Improving Cancer Services Through Patient Involvement

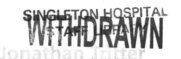
Norma Daykin
Simon Evans
and
Michail Sanidas

Foreword by

Professor Mike Richards
National Cancer Director

Radcliffe Medical Press

Radcliffe Medical Press Ltd
18 Marcham Road
Abingdon
Oxon OX14 1AA
United Kingdom

www.radcliffe-oxford.com
The Radcliffe Medical Press electronic catalogue and online ordering facility.
Direct sales to anywhere in the world.

British Library Cataloguing in Publication Data

A catalogue record for this book is available from the British Library.

ISBN 1 85775 844 7

Typeset by Advance Typesetting Ltd, Oxfordshire
Printed and bound by TJ International Ltd, Padstow, Cornwall

Contents

Foreword

The Calman–Hine Report (1995) set out seven key principles which should govern the provision of cancer care. One of these principles is that 'the development of cancer services should be patient centred and should take account of patients' families and carers' views and preferences as well as those of professionals involved in cancer care'. This principle was re-emphasised in the *NHS Cancer Plan* (2000) which made it clear that 'at a local level cancer networks will be expected to take account of the views of patients and carers when planning services'.

The principle of incorporating users' views in the development and evaluation of NHS services is much more widely accepted now than it was even a decade ago. However, until now there has been relatively little guidance on good practice relating to user involvement.

This toolkit for user involvement has been derived from the extensive experience of one cancer network which has pioneered the involvement of users in developing and evaluating services. The toolkit is the product of a major collaboration over several years between professionals, patients and carers within the Avon, Somerset and Wiltshire cancer network. This collaboration has been supported by two universities and two national charities and by a grant from the Department of Health.

The authors make a strong case for user involvement being seen as a continuous cycle rather than as a one-off activity. The individual steps in the 'user involvement cycle' are set out in separate chapters. Each chapter in Part 1 of the toolkit highlights key issues and provides practical examples derived from the experience in Avon, Somerset and Wiltshire.

Part 2 of the toolkit provides detailed advice on the tools and methods which are available to make user involvement a reality. The authors rightly emphasise that those who wish to establish user involvement processes do not need to start from scratch, but can use and adapt well tried and tested methods.

The toolkit is extremely readable and will, I believe, be of great value to all those who are trying to develop user involvement in cancer services in the UK. The toolkit will be of interest to people working at the level of the cancer team, the whole organisation (e.g. NHS Trust or Voluntary Hospice) and the cancer network. The experience should also be of value to those working in fields other than cancer.

Professor Mike Richards
National Cancer Director
September 2003

About the authors

Jonathan Q Tritter
Lecturer in Medical Sociology
Department of Sociology
University of Warwick

Norma Daykin
Reader in Health, Community and Policy Studies
University of the West of England, Bristol

Simon Evans
Research Fellow
Faculty of Health and Social Care
University of the West of England, Bristol
Research Facilitator
Avon and Wiltshire Mental Health Partnership NHS Trust

Michail Sanidas
Macmillan Project Officer for User Involvement
Avon, Somerset and Wiltshire Cancer Services

Acknowledgements

We would like to acknowledge the Department of Health (grant 370051) which funded the research on which we based this *Toolkit*.

The *Toolkit* is the product of the collaborative work of the Best Practice in Evaluating and Developing User Involvement Research Project Team. The text was primarily drafted by Norma Daykin (University of the West of England), Simon Evans (University of the West of England), Michail Sanidas (Avon, Somerset and Wiltshire Cancer Services) and Jonathan Tritter (University of Warwick), who also co-ordinated the work.

The other members of the Project Steering Group, namely Victor Barley (Avon, Somerset and Wiltshire Cancer Services), Judith McNeill (Macmillan Cancer Care), Nigel Palmer (User Representative), James Rimmer (Avon, Somerset and Wiltshire Cancer Services) and Pat Turton (Bristol Cancer Help Centre), provided essential input on content and style, as well as keen editorial advice, and without them the *Toolkit* could not have been written. We are also grateful to Sarah Mitchard and Ruth Newport, who were involved during the early stages of the project and whose help in gathering information was invaluable.

Many other people also contributed to the development of the *Toolkit*. In particular, we would like to thank Christine Farrell for her guidance and input at many stages of the research. We would also like to thank the following experts who contributed to the seminar on *Developing a Toolkit for Building User Involvement Systems in Cancer Services* in May 2002: Denise Adcock, Jo Allen, Ros Ashley, Jane Bradburn, Sarah Buckland, Katie Burall, Marj Clark, Cathryn Havard, Tracey Jones, Helen Langton, Helen Lester, Ingrid Marshall, Louise North, Michael Shepherd, Emma Sims, Pat Taylor, Patricia Vernon, Isobel Woolley and Annie Young. Their input was essential for helping to ensure the quality and utility of what we have produced.

Finally, we would like to thank all of the users – patients, carers and health professionals – who helped us to understand what would make user involvement work best. They have helped to ensure that cancer services for everybody are evaluated, developed and improved.

PART 1

The user involvement cycle

Introducing the *Toolkit*

In this section, we:

- set out the aims of this *Toolkit* and explain who it is for
- explain how we developed this *Toolkit* as part of a three-year study funded by the Department of Health
- provide a brief overview of the contents of the *Toolkit* and guidance on how to use it
- look at the concept of user involvement
- introduce a *cycle of user involvement* as a way of thinking systematically about the process of user involvement
- discuss direct and indirect user involvement
- outline the national policy background to user involvement in health services in the UK.

Aims

Avon, Somerset and Wiltshire Cancer Services (ASWCS) produced this *Toolkit* primarily for people in the NHS who provide and deliver health services. The aim is to help them to involve the people who use health services in the evaluation and development of those services.

We set out a range of ideas, practical suggestions and examples of methods of user involvement that have been tried and tested. We hope that the *Toolkit* will help people to improve the quality of care both in cancer services and in other areas of healthcare.

We designed the *Toolkit* to help people to think about user involvement in cancer services. This is now especially important as health professionals and managers are being asked to demonstrate that they involve service users in planning services.

Who is the *Toolkit* for?

Current policies, discussed below, make it clear that cancer networks,* multidisciplinary teams, primary care teams and all NHS cancer services

---

*Cancer networks are regional collaborations between strategic health authorities, NHS trusts, primary care organisations, hospices, service users, local authorities and voluntary organisations. They aim to improve the quality of cancer services.

are responsible for developing user involvement in service evaluation and delivery. Although various national initiatives have been set up for user involvement, action at local level is also important.

Consultants, specialist nurses, radiographers, managers and others all need to involve users in decisions about how to develop services. The *Toolkit* aims to help with different types of user involvement as part of service evaluation and development. In particular, it will help cancer networks and multidisciplinary teams to act on the *NHS Cancer Plan* (Department of Health, 2000a) recommendations to improve the patient experience, in line with guidance from the Cancer Collaborative.*

We also hope that a wider range of individuals will find this *Toolkit* useful. Educationalists, researchers, user groups and others seeking to get involved or learn more about user involvement in cancer services will find much useful information within these pages.

Developing the *Toolkit*: the ASWCS Project

We developed the *Toolkit* from a project on developing and evaluating user involvement in cancer services. This project took place in Avon, Somerset and Wiltshire Cancer Services (ASWCS), one of 34 cancer networks in the UK that were established following the recommendations of the 1995 Calman–Hine report (Department of Health, 1995). It was a three-year study of *best practice in developing and evaluating user involvement in cancer services*. The Department of Health Policy Research Programme funded the study as part of the Health in Partnership Initiative. It was a collaboration between ASWCS, Warwick University, the University of the West of England (Bristol) together with one local and one national voluntary organisation.

The project was based across the three health authorities (Avon, Somerset and Wiltshire) that form the ASWCS network. ASWCS covers a population of 2.05 million people and includes seven NHS trusts, six hospices and twelve primary care trusts. Around 22% of the population is over 60 years of age, and approximately 20 000 new cases of cancer are diagnosed annually.

The project began with a mapping exercise to identify current mechanisms of user involvement. The next stage was to develop a consensus statement on the role and extent of user involvement in cancer services. We based the consensus statement on the views of users, health professionals and voluntary organisations. It is reproduced in Part 2: Sections 3E and 3F.

---

*The Cancer Collaborative is an NHS programme across each of the 34 cancer networks. It aims to support local clinical teams in looking at their service and making significant improvements for patients by redesigning the way in which cancer care is delivered.

In order to explore good practice in user involvement, we carried out in-depth case studies of three hospital NHS trusts. These focused on definitions and experiences of user involvement in the multidisciplinary teams that care for people with breast, colorectal, lung and prostate cancer, as well as in the palliative care teams.

We conducted in-depth interviews with cancer patients from a range of backgrounds in order to document users' experiences and find out what users thought about the involvement they had experienced. We used the results of this research to design a questionnaire for a survey of over 600 patients, exploring their experiences and satisfaction with user involvement.

This *Toolkit* brings together the different types of evidence that were gathered during the research. The examples we use throughout the *Toolkit* are real and based on our own experience. We have included the research tools that were validated during the course of the project in Part 2, Section 3. You can use these as they stand or adapt them to suit your particular needs. Many other methods and tools exist, and an overview of some of these is provided in Part 2, Section 1.

How to use the *Toolkit*

Overview of contents

This *Toolkit* is presented in two parts:

- Part 1 – the user involvement cycle
- Part 2 – tools and methods.

Part 1: the user involvement cycle

Part 1 is organised in ten sections. The first eight sections focus on the *cycle of user involvement*, which we introduce below. Sections 2 to 8 each consider a different stage of the cycle, exploring the strategies and resources that are needed at each stage. Each section contains a brief discussion of the issues that arise at a particular stage. Sections 9 and 10 focus on ongoing issues that arise throughout the cycle, namely education and training, and ethical issues. Research has shown that user involvement is unlikely to occur without support and training for professionals, and for this reason Section 9 explores the issues that are involved in providing interprofessional education for user involvement. Section 10 explores the ethical issues associated with user involvement, including a discussion of the role of ethics committees.

In each section we use examples and case studies to illustrate key issues, and we refer you to Part 2 for further details on how to use particular methods.

Each section ends with a series of frequently asked questions. These are questions that arose during the course of our project, and we have provided a brief discussion to help you to think around the issues. We have also provided recommendations for further reading for those who wish to explore particular issues in more depth.

Part 2: tools and methods

Part 2 is organised in three sections. Section 1 provides a comprehensive overview and glossary of tools and methods for user involvement activities in the health services. In Section 2, we provide detailed descriptions of nine useful methods and procedures, namely methods for developing consensus, questionnaires, focus groups, interviews, setting up a website, producing a newsletter, running a workshop, and setting up a user involvement training programme. This is followed in Section 3 by details of the research tools and methods that we have found particularly helpful and used successfully in our project.

Using the *Toolkit*

There are many different ways of using this *Toolkit*. Some people will want to read it from cover to cover, perhaps as a part of a user involvement training programme. Others might use particular sections to help with a specific user involvement activity or to develop a user involvement partnership.

People in many different roles – including consultants, specialist nurses, radiographers and managers – will have different needs in relation to user involvement. Although people with different roles may seek different types of information, sections of this *Toolkit* should be valuable for everyone who is seeking to involve service users in decisions about how to improve and develop services.

Table 1.1 opposite shows a map of the contents of Part 1 of the *Toolkit*, identifying different pathways through it to help you to find the sections that you need. For example, if you want to find out how to set up a user involvement system, Sections 1, 2, 7, 8 and 9 will be particularly useful.

User involvement

The user involvement cycle

Throughout this *Toolkit* we emphasise the need for involving service users in a systematic way and building user involvement practices into the way in which you organise and deliver care.

Table 1.1:   Pathways through Part 1 of the user involvement *Toolkit*

Your needs	Sections in the Toolkit									
	Section 1 Introducing the *Toolkit*	Section 2 Identifying service users	Section 3 Defining the aims of user involvement	Section 4 Mapping user involvement	Section 5 Documenting service user experiences	Section 6 Involving users in service evaluation and development	Section 7 Developing and evaluating a user involvement system	Section 8 Implementation and dissemination	Section 9 Professional education and training for user involvement	Section 10 Ethical issues
Finding out more about user involvement	✓✓	✓✓	✓✓				✓		✓	✓
As part of a training programme	✓✓	✓✓	✓✓	✓✓	✓✓	✓✓	✓✓	✓✓	✓✓	✓✓
'One-off' user involvement exercise	✓✓	✓✓	✓✓	✓	✓✓	✓✓		✓	✓	✓✓
Developing a user involvement system	✓✓	✓✓	✓	✓	✓	✓	✓✓	✓✓	✓	✓✓
Considering methods of user involvement	✓✓	✓		✓✓	✓✓	✓✓	✓			✓✓
Evaluating user involvement	✓✓	✓	✓		✓✓	✓✓	✓✓	✓	✓✓	✓✓

✓✓, most important; ✓, useful but not essential.

Building a system of user involvement for evaluating and developing services is complicated and takes time. The cycle of user involvement (*see* Figure 1.1) presents a way of thinking systematically about the process of user involvement.

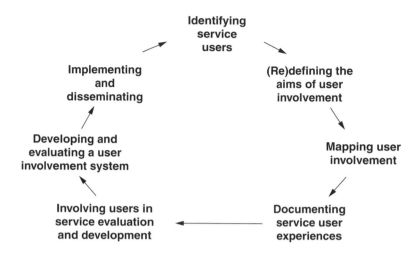

Figure 1.1 Cycle of user involvement.

User involvement should not be a 'one-off' activity, but rather it should be part of an integrated system. A systematic approach helps to ensure that changes which are made because of users' views are evaluated.

Undertaking a specific user involvement activity (e.g. a carer satisfaction questionnaire about a cancer information centre) is likely to tell you something about how the carers who completed the survey felt about the information provision at that time. It might suggest things that you could do to improve it. However, you need to go round the cycle again to repeat the survey in order to check that the changes that have been put in place bring real improvements. Thus repetition holds the key to ensuring that changes inspired by users' views actually make the service better. Without repetition there is no way to be certain that user involvement is being successfully used for service development.

The different components of the cycle relate to one another and each phase of the process (or cycle) builds on the last phase and leads to the next one. This cyclic process helps to ensure that you conduct user involvement activities in a planned way that links directly to changes in service organisation and provision, and that service users continually evaluate these changes.

Direct and indirect user involvement

A distinction can be made between direct and indirect forms of involvement.

Direct involvement

Direct involvement occurs when service users are involved directly in decision making. Users can be directly involved in a wide range of decisions – not just those about their own treatment (although this is of course important), but also decisions about service development, including the type of service offered, improvements that are needed and the use of resources.

A variety of methods are available for involving users directly in decision making, many of which we discuss in the *Toolkit*. For example, many organisations have user representatives on steering groups and committees at different levels within the organisation. Others have special *user involvement groups* that advise on policy development and decision making across the organisation. These groups typically have members drawn from professional groups and service users, and they can provide a useful forum for bringing together different experiences, perspectives and expertise.

Indirect involvement

Indirect involvement is more limited than direct involvement, but it can still be very useful. Indirect involvement often involves information gathering by professionals in order to inform service delivery and development. Although professionals may seek and act upon users' feedback, in indirect involvement professionals make the final decisions.

One of the difficulties with indirect involvement is that professionals can choose to ignore users' feedback if they do not think it is appropriate. As a result, users who have contributed to the process may feel frustrated.

In this *Toolkit* we emphasise the importance of feedback and dissemination as a key part of the user involvement cycle, whatever form of user involvement has taken place and regardless of the decisions made.

User involvement: the UK policy context

Public and patient participation has a long history in the UK, and is linked to issues of democratic accountability and consumerism. This history extends from the establishment of Community Health Councils in 1974, with an increased emphasis on user involvement given by The Patient's Charter

(Department of Health, 1991) and the *Local Voices* White Paper (Sykes *et al.*, 1992). In 1996, the publication of a discussion paper entitled *Patient Partnership: Building a Collaborative Strategy* made clear the importance of gathering information from users (patients and carers) on their 'perception of individual services and their views on wider priorities' (Department of Health, NHS Executive, 1996: 3).

More recently, the publication of *Patient and Public Involvement in the New NHS* (Department of Health, 1999) and *The NHS Plan* (Department of Health, 2000b) have placed user involvement at the centre of the development and evaluation of services:

> NHS care has to be shaped around the convenience and concerns of patients. To bring this about, patients must have more say in their own treatment and more influence over the way the NHS works.
>
> (Department of Health, 2000b: 88)

The Commission for Health Improvement now assesses the nature, extent and quality of user involvement in their clinical governance reviews.

User involvement is also increasingly important in cancer services. In 1995, the publication of the Calman–Hine Report, *A Policy Framework for Commissioning Cancer Services* (Department of Health, 1995), set the tone for the reform and reorganisation of cancer care and established the ideal of patient-centred cancer services. More recently, this approach has been developed in the *NHS Cancer Plan* (Department of Health, 2000a), which states that cancer networks need to take account of the views of patients and carers when planning services (Department of Health, 2000a: 69). Service users are also involved in the Cancer Information and Advisory Group and the Cancer Taskforce.

The recent passage of the Health and Social Care Act and the NHS Reform and Health Care Professions Bill reaffirm and strengthen the role that users should play. They led to the development of Patients' Forums in every NHS trust and the establishment of a new national body to oversee them, namely the Commission for Patient and Public Involvement in Health. The duty of all NHS trusts and health authorities to consult with and involve users is now enshrined in law. As the Health and Social Care Act states in section 11:

> It is the duty of every body to which this section applies to make arrangements with a view to securing, as respects health services for which it is responsible, that persons to whom those services are being or may be provided are, directly or through representatives, involved in and consulted on (a) the planning of the provision of those services, (b) the development and consideration of proposals for changes in the way those services are provided, and (c) decisions to be made by that body affecting the operation of those services.
>
> This section applies to (a) health authorities, (b) primary care trusts, and (c) NHS trusts.

Implementing user involvement policies

> At a local level, cancer networks will be expected to take account of the views of patients and carers when planning services.
>
> (Department of Health, 2000a: 7.19)

The *NHS Cancer Plan* requires cancer networks to ensure that patients and carers have their say in the development and delivery of cancer services. This is partly to be achieved through national initiatives such as the Cancer Services Collaborative, Supportive Care Networks* and Cancer Partnership Project[+] funding for developing user involvement in cancer networks. Local initiatives are also important, including surveys, user groups and other participation events.

The Cancer Services Collaborative has the clear aim of building patient experience into the improvement of cancer services. As with all areas of the Collaborative, this improvement should be based on clear evaluation and the existence of a system for implementing suggested improvements. Supportive care networks are being set up within cancer networks to look at the psychological, social and spiritual needs of cancer patients. These groupings are developing alongside but distinct from palliative care[‡] networks. User involvement is key to the success of the supportive care networks, and many of the issues arising from them focus on the information needs of patients and carers.

The Cancer Partnership Project has made funding available for a central resource – often a person – within each cancer network team to support user involvement. In addition, Macmillan Cancer Relief has supported the project with up to £5000 per network to fund user-led initiatives.

These initiatives and others give cancer networks, multidisciplinary teams, primary care teams and all NHS cancer services a focus for developing user involvement. The policies outlined above are being actively supported and funded with the aim of greater patient and public participation. This *Toolkit* aims to support these developments and give those interested in taking them forward some suggestions and examples.

---

*Supportive care networks are established alongside cancer networks to provide evidence-based recommendations on how best to ensure that patients receive high-quality information, communication, symptom control, and psychological, social and spiritual support.

[+]The Cancer Partnership Project is an initiative to support user involvement within cancer networks, led by Macmillan Cancer Relief and the Department of Health.

[‡]Palliative care services are for people who are terminally ill, usually to reduce pain or to help them to live longer.

References

- Department of Health (1991) *The Patient's Charter.* HMSO, London.
- Department of Health (1995) *Improving the Quality of Cancer Services. A Report by the Expert Advisory Group on Cancer to the Chief Medical Officers of England and Wales.* HMSO, London.
- Department of Health and the Welsh Office (1995) *A Policy Framework for Commissioning Cancer Services: A Report by the Expert Advisory Group on Cancer to the Chief Medical Officers of England and Wales. Guidance for Purchasers and Providers of Cancer Services.* Department of Health, London.
- Department of Health, NHS Executive (1996) *Patient Partnership: building a collaborative strategy.* Department of Health, Leeds.
- Department of Health (1999) *Patient and Public Involvement in the New NHS.* Department of Health, London.
- Department of Health (2000a) *The NHS Cancer Plan;* www.doh.gov.uk/cancer/cancerplan.htm
- Department of Health (2000b) *The NHS Plan: a plan for investment, a plan for reform.* Department of Health, Leeds; www.doh.gov.uk/nhsplan
- Sykes W, Collins M, Hunter DJ, Popay J and Williams G (1992) *Listening to Local Voices: a guide to research methods.* Nuffield Institute for Health Services Studies, University of Leeds, Leeds.

Further reading

- Arnstein S (1969) A ladder of citizen participation. *J Am Inst Planners.* **35**: 216–24.
- Clarke R (2000) *Public and Patient Involvement in England, Scotland and Northern Ireland: what works?* Institute for Public Policy Research, London.
- Commission for Health Improvement (2002) *'Nothing About Us Without Us': the patient and public strategy for CHI.* Commission for Health Improvement, London; www.chi.nhs.uk/patients/strategy.pdf
- Department of Health, Flinders University, and the South Australian Community Health Research Unit (2000) *Improving Health Services Through Consumer Participation.* Department of Health, Flinders University, and the South Australian Community Health Research Unit, Adelaide; http://nrccph.latrobe.edu.au/
- NHS Confederation (2002) *Getting Closer: a guide to partnerships in new health policy.* NHS Confederation, London.
- NHS Modernisation Agency (2000) *Improvement Leaders' Guide to Involving Patients and Carers;* www.modern.nhs.uk/improvementguides/reading/involving_patients.pdf
- Office for Public Management and National Assembly for Wales (2001) *Signposts: a practical guide to public and patient involvement in Wales.* National Assembly for Wales, Cardiff; www.wales.gov.uk/subihealth/content/nhs/signposts/signposts-e.pdf
- Scottish Consumer Council (1999) *Designed to Involve: public involvement in the new primary care structures;* www.designedtoinvolve.org.uk/homt.htm
- Simpson EL, House AO and Barkhamb M (2002) *A Guide to Involving Users, Ex-Users and Carers in Mental Health Service Planning, Delivery or Research: a health technology approach.* University of Leeds; www.leeds.ac.uk/medicine/divisions/psychiatry/research/guidebook.htm

SECTION 2

Identifying service users

This section focuses on the *identifying service users* stage of the cycle of user involvement.

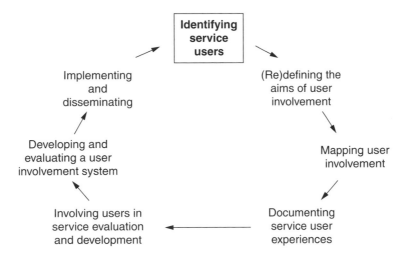

Cycle of user involvement.

In this section, we discuss:

- the rationale for user involvement
- the range of people who may be defined as 'service users'
- ways of identifying and involving a diverse range of users, including hard-to-reach groups
- identifying and approaching service users for 'one-off' involvement exercises and for user involvement partnerships
- using the media to recruit service users
- issues of user representation
- sampling – deciding who to include, sampling methods and strategies
- a summary checklist
- frequently asked questions.

Summary of key issues

- The rationale for user involvement is that it is a prerequisite for developing patient-centred services.
- There are different methods for defining users. The definition of who to include in service development can depend on many factors, including the particular objectives of a project. There is a surprising lack of agreement on this issue – users can be defined either relatively narrowly as current patients and their carers, or broadly to include the public as taxpayers or potential service users. Some definitions of user involvement also include professional stakeholders.
- We do not suggest that there are right or wrong answers to the question 'Who are users?', but we do argue that it is important to be clear about the reasons why particular users are targeted in service evaluation and development.
- We suggest that the process of documenting users' views and involving users in decision making is likely to be strengthened by including as diverse a range of views as possible.
- Different types of user involvement activity show how the objectives of each activity influence one's definition of users. Activities range from mapping existing user involvement and finding out what users think about this, to involving individual users in decision making as members or representatives of committees, project steering groups and other bodies.
- Issues that arise in particular when considering the role of users as either informants or representatives include the need to involve hard-to-reach groups. We suggest strategies for this.
- There are many issues to consider with regard to user representation and sampling. Sampling is a relatively formal procedure associated with research. Although most user involvement activities are considered to be part of service development rather than research, it is still important that these are as accurate, objective and inclusive as possible. We outline six different sampling strategies.
- The defining of service users cannot easily be considered in isolation from other issues. Links and overlaps are shown in the *frequently asked questions* at the end of this section.

Rationale for user involvement

The development of user involvement in cancer services was driven by the 1995 Calman–Hine Report, which led to the reorganisation of cancer services in England and Wales. One of the general principles advocated by the report was as follows:

> The development of cancer services should be patient-centred and should take account of patients', families' and carers' views and preferences as well as those of professionals involved in cancer care. Individuals' perceptions of their needs may differ from those of the professionals. Good communication between professionals and patients is especially important.

> (Department of Health, 1995: 6)

User involvement is a prerequisite for developing patient-centred cancer services. Developing a user involvement system raises a number of questions, including which service users to involve, how to elicit users' views and how to communicate effectively with service users.

Identifying and approaching service users

The definition of users may depend on the type of service development you wish to undertake. For instance, if you were evaluating a 'hospice at home' service, you would involve different groups of people compared with those you would involve if you were reviewing information provided in a breast care clinic.

Defining service users and stakeholders

There is a surprising lack of agreement about who service users are. They may be patients, carers or members of support groups and voluntary organisations who represent them. They may be current, past or even potential service users. Healthcare professionals, as providers or commissioners of services, are also stakeholders and are sometimes considered to be users in their own right.

Users and stakeholders may be:

- patients and carers
- potential service users
- the general public
- members of voluntary organisations
- healthcare professionals as commissioners of services
- service providers.

As part of the ASWCS research project, health professionals and service users were asked to define who cancer services users are. The results of this exercise are shown in Figure 2.1. Most people agree that patients should be involved in the evaluation, planning and development of cancer services. However, there is much less agreement about whether voluntary organisations and the public should be involved. This does not imply that it is wrong to involve these groups, but it is important to recognise that there may be resistance to involving them.

This means that it is important to be clear why you want to get different groups of people involved. Clearly defined aims influence the way in which users are defined, as well as the ways of getting them involved.

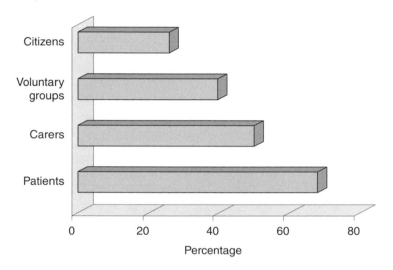

Figure 2.1 Percentage of respondents who strongly agree that different groups are users of cancer services.

Capturing a diversity of users and users' views

Clearly, the different experiences that people have may mean that their views will vary and possibly conflict with each other.

In order to learn from a broad range of experiences, user involvement should aim to capture as wide a range of views as possible. This means that it is important to involve different categories of users. Some of the key questions to ask when you are deciding who to involve include the following.

• Who directly uses the service?
• Who needs to communicate with the service providers?
• Who is likely to use the service in the future?
• Are there any support groups or voluntary organisations that relate to this service?

It is important to be sensitive to people who may encounter difficulties in making their views known, and to consider how to ensure that you include them. This may include people who, for example:

- are disabled
- do not have easy access to transport
- have communication or reading difficulties
- are not fluent in English.

Sometimes the hard-to-reach users can be approached through voluntary or community organisations that work with them. You should consider how to contact and develop relationships with these organisations in order to involve them and understand the needs of the full range of service users.

Thinking about categories of users: documentation of user experience

The documentation of users' experiences is one of the first steps in evaluating and developing patient-centred services. (In this *Toolkit* we provide some examples of this process, showing how different types of questions can only be answered by involving different types of users.)

Documenting users' experiences can sometimes be a useful 'one-off' exercise, although ideally this should be integrated into a broader user involvement partnership. Even when undertaking one-off exercises it is important to give feedback to those who have taken part, otherwise users may feel that their views have not been acted upon.

'One-off' user involvement exercises

Imagine that a community liaison officer wants to find out about the image and understanding of the hospice that she serves. She would need to involve a broad range of users, including people living in the local area. She could use a range of methods. For example, a *survey of local people* might provide a snapshot of how people perceive the hospice. She could also hold an *open public meeting*, at which community leaders could be invited to talk about the importance of the hospice.

A *mapping exercise* is another example of a user involvement exercise. This can be used to document users' experiences or to collect information about what activities professionals are involved in at a given time. It may be a one-off exercise or it can be incorporated into a broader partnership or user involvement cycle.

We used a mapping exercise in the ASWCS research study. One of our aims was to find out what definitions of user involvement existed within the network. We also sought to determine what methods were currently being used to involve service users. The ASWCS exercise is set out below, and a discussion of how to undertake a mapping exercise is provided in Part 2, Section 2C.

Example: mapping user involvement in ASWCS

The ASWCS mapping exercise sought to gain an overview of user involvement across the statutory and voluntary sectors in Avon, Somerset and Wiltshire.

The first step was to decide who should be included. It was important to include all organisations operating within the catchment area of the cancer network, and these were identified from the cancer network database.

The following table provides a breakdown of the mapping exercise sample and illustrates the different categories of professionals and service user groups that we accessed.

Type of organisation	Person receiving questionnaire
NHS trust	Chief Executive
	Public involvement lead
	Cancer Manager
	Clinical Governance Director
	Research and Development Coordinator
Health authority	Cancer lead
	Public involvement lead
Hospices	Chief Executive or General Manager
Primary care groups	Chairperson
Community health councils	Chief Officer
Social Services	Director
Voluntary and support groups	Organisations run by professionals
	Organisations run by users
	Non-cancer-specific organisations (carer support)

Selecting users for user involvement partnerships

As well as one-off exercises, user involvement requires longer-term relationships between professionals and users. This raises particular questions about who the appropriate users and stakeholders are, and requires effective methods of involving them.

These longer-term partnerships can take many forms. One example is the involvement of user representatives in advisory and decision-making committees within organisations. This raises questions about the recruitment and selection of users as well as about the role, expectations and needs of user representatives.

In the case study below, we describe an example of this process, based on our own experience of involving users (patients and carers) as members of the steering group of our study. We discuss the recruitment and selection process that we used, the selection criteria and role description. We also describe the support we provided to the involved users.

Case study: involving users in ASWCS project steering group

Selection process and criteria
The steering group sought to include two user representatives as members of the project advisory group. This was a relatively long-term role, with the possibility of being involved for up to three years as well as taking part in follow-up activities after the project was complete. We felt that it was important not to exclude service users who were unable to offer such a long-term commitment, and to try to incorporate as wide a range of user views as possible.

The selection criteria and process were designed to address these concerns. We sought to generate a broad pool of interested users who were willing to participate in the project for a minimum of two months. This allowed individuals to take turns participating in the steering group, with each user agreeing to be present for at least two consecutive meetings. In order to provide continuity, the terms of the involved users would overlap. It was also important to provide support for the user representatives as well as accountability, so we asked the pool of users to serve as a reference and support group.

We based the selection of user members of the steering group on criteria designed to enable individuals to contribute effectively to the work of the project. Following discussion and consultation with members of ASWCS standing user involvement group, we decided to exclude individuals with a recent diagnosis of cancer on the grounds that they might find the process traumatic. We wanted to recruit people who could give a commitment to attend monthly meetings and who were in communication with other cancer service users (e.g. as members of a support group). Therefore we used the following selection criteria.

- The time since diagnosis of cancer must be more than one year and less than ten years (after ten years users are discharged from routine follow-up).
- Members should potentially be able to attend steering group meetings every month (health and holidays permitting).

continued overleaf

- Users must be in contact with other cancer service users (via support group, user group or similar).
- Users will have support from one member of the project team, and they will decide who this will be.

Recruiting users

We felt that it was important to offer a wide range of service users the opportunity to be involved. In order to include those who already had experience of involvement, we informed members of the cancer network's standing user involvement group about the opportunity. To include a wider group, we also advertised in the local press. We issued a press release asking for volunteers, followed by interviews given by members of our project team on two local radio programmes.

People who were interested in finding out more were given a telephone number and an opportunity to discuss the research and the role of steering group members with an existing member. We sent written information about the project and a role description (see below) to those who were interested in becoming more involved. We asked them to send us a letter giving some information about themselves as a service user and their interest in participating in the project.

Role description

The group agreed that the role of the user member was to draw on their own experiences and those of other cancer service users to help to ensure that users' needs were considered throughout the research project. The user members would play a full part in project meetings and have a say in decisions about the project that was equal to that of the professionals.

The role description for the user member of the project steering group was as follows:

- contributing to the discussions and decisions of the steering group
- preparing for the meetings by reading through the agenda and accompanying papers and consulting with others where appropriate
- attending the monthly steering group meetings
- user members are free to leave the steering group at any time.

Supporting the user member

We considered that user members would need different types of support. Initially, we sent interested users the relevant project information by post and offered an opportunity to talk to a member of the steering group. Prior to the first attendance at a steering group meeting, an informal meeting was arranged with one of the researchers in order to answer any service users' questions.

continued opposite

User members received a copy of the agenda together with all accompanying papers by email or post. A member of the team was always available for a pre-meeting briefing 45 minutes before each meeting, and spoke on the phone to user members at least once a month. We also discussed specific exit strategies for those users who wanted to end their participation. We provided opportunities for informal discussion with members of the steering group. In addition, we offered the user a referral for counselling or discussion with medical staff.

Financial considerations

Involvement often bears financial and other costs for users. Furthermore, professionals who are taking part in user involvement are paid for their time, and this can contribute to unequal relationships between professionals and users who are often volunteers. We sought to address this situation by paying each user member an honorarium.

The figure agreed was £50 per month, plus travel expenses. The honorarium was in recognition of pre- and post-meeting activities, reading documents and providing feedback and comments. We felt that this served to acknowledge users' time and expertise, but was not large enough to serve as an independent incentive for taking part.

Any additional activities in which the user member wanted to take part, such as conference participation, were funded if they were clearly and directly linked to the work of the project.

Key points

This discussion has highlighted a range of factors to consider when planning effective user involvement. These are summarised below.

- Make sure that you make it clear why you want to get service users involved.
- Develop clear terms of reference, person and role descriptions for involved users.
- Draw up a list of key organisations that you need to contact (search the Internet, and contact national groups such as Cancerlink or the Patient Forum or local groups such as the Community Service Volunteers).
- Check whether there is a local user liaison group.
- Convey your message in an accessible manner. Consider presenting your information in plain English and other formats such as ASCII.
- Make imaginative use of the different media. Use posters, newsletters, press releases and the Internet (an example of a press release is provided below).
- Consider the training needs of involved users.

continued overleaf

- Help users to prepare for involvement (e.g. by giving an overview of the project, its contribution to the NHS and the work of a given committee).
- Create a clear and transparent recruitment and selection process.
- Provide opportunities for support, accountability and communication between user members and other user groups.
- Provide adequate resources to support user involvement.
- Offer ongoing support (e.g. through a buddy system), to user representatives.

Using the media to recruit service users

The press and local radio/television can be cheap and effective ways of reaching a wide local audience. If your organisation has an information office, they may be able to help with this. Below is a sample press release aimed at recruiting service users.

Example of a press release

Do you have experience of cancer, either as a patient or as a carer of someone with cancer? If so, you might be interested in taking part in a research project looking at how users of cancer services can be involved in developing and changing services.

Users of cancer services are already involved in the research project informally in many different ways. For example, service users have spoken about their experiences by taking part in focus groups. Now the project is looking for volunteers to be members of the Steering Group that helps to direct the project. The project needs two representatives on the Steering Group at any one time, and if there were more than two volunteers a pool of representatives would be set up. The Steering Group meets monthly.

You do not need to have experience of formal meetings like a Steering Group to take part. It is your experience of coping with cancer that is very valuable to the project. You would be supported in your role by a named member of the group, who would go through the agenda with you before each meeting. A payment would be made to cover your attendance at the meeting and also all necessary activities outside of the meeting, such as reading the material for the meeting. Expenses like travel costs or childcare would also be paid.

If you think you can help, please get in touch. You need to have experience of cancer either as a patient or as a carer, with a cancer that has been diagnosed at least a year ago, but within the past five years. If you are interested, contact AN Other for a chat at Cancer Services on xxxxx, or email her at an.other@aswcs.nhs.uk

User representation

Are service users representative?

A key aspect of involving users concerns how representative they are of all the people who use the services.

If users are seen as 'unrepresentative', then the value of their input is sometimes diminished (although it is worth noting that it is not generally expected that professional members of committees would be representative in the same way). Users, like professionals, will provide input based on their own experience. Being too concerned that involved users are representative, or that all possible users are involved, can get in the way of ensuring that users' views are being used to shape services.

Including people who are ill or hard to reach

It is important to consider ways of including people from hard-to-reach or marginalised groups who may be less likely than others to get involved. Excluding these groups will result in the loss of valuable information about services. It would be easy to approach the people that local health services often work with, but their views are likely to have been shaped by long experience of involvement.

Involving users from hard-to-reach groups is often seen as particularly challenging. If conventional approaches have been unsuccessful in the past, they are unlikely to work in the future, and new methods may be needed. For example, involvement of ethnic minorities in cancer-specific projects may be rare, but it is possible to liaise with general health and community support projects to find out about people's experiences of cancer and other services.

One useful approach is to involve people from the voluntary sector. There is a wide range of local, regional and national voluntary organisations that provide services and support for people with cancer. These organisations may be able to help with accessing diverse user perspectives as well as identifying individuals who may wish to get involved.

If you ask for help from voluntary organisations, you should consider the time and money constraints that these groups face. You should also consider possible 'consultation fatigue' when the same groups or individuals are repeatedly approached.

You should try not to exclude anyone who wishes to be involved. Not everyone wants to get involved, and some people may wish to be involved only at certain points in their life or during the course of their illness. You should not use someone's health condition as a reason not to consult them. There are good examples of very ill people, including those in hospices, actively seeking to be involved and successfully participating in user involvement activities.

Sampling

Deciding who to include in your sample

You cannot involve all people all of the time for every issue, so it is important to consider carefully who you do involve in order to obtain information that is as valid, accurate and representative as possible, depending on the objectives that you want to achieve. This is the basis of sampling, on which some user involvement activities depend.

Once you have identified the groups and individuals you wish to involve as users, you need to consider which of them you will ask to take part in your user involvement exercise. Ideally, you would want all of them to participate, but that is unlikely to be possible or practicable. Instead, you want as many of the 'right' users to be involved as possible – this group forms the sample of users to be included. It is also important that you include the full range of people who make up your target group in your sample, such as the following:

- men and women
- people who have families and those who are single
- people from different socio-economic and ethnic backgrounds
- people with disabilities.

If the full range of different types of users is involved, and in the same proportion as they are in the broader population, you will maximise the likelihood that the views of your participants represent those of all service users.

There are different ways to think about recruiting the 'right' types of users and the implications that this has for the conclusions you reach.

Sampling allows you to study some of, rather than all of, the users who are of interest, while drawing valid conclusions about all of those in a specific user category. In a user involvement context, sampling refers to those who 'represent' the public.

Choosing a sampling method

You need to balance three factors when selecting a sampling method:

- the *purpose* of the study – what you want to learn and why
- the *accuracy* of the sample – involving only a few people from the 'right' group of users may give you a perspective that does not reflect the views of most of the group
- The *cost* in time, money and effort.

The following factors are also important:

- the *size* of the sample – the smaller the group taking part, the less representative it is of the overall population being studied
- the *socio-economic group* – people of higher socio-economic status are more able to bear the costs of involvement and may therefore tend to be more likely to be willing to participate. This means that they can be over-represented in user involvement activities.

It may be useful to seek expert statistical advice on how to construct your sample, particularly if you need to make power calculations* or you want your results to be statistically significant.[†]

Sampling strategies

Below we outline six different sampling strategies. Each of these has pros and cons, and the choice of strategy may also depend on the question that you want to answer. In addition, it is worth remembering that no matter how carefully you construct your sample, people may still refuse to be involved.

Census

A census is often the best method when there is a need for minimal error. Data are collected from every member of some specified population. For example, the cancer registry collects information about all new cancer cases in a given area.

Self-selected sample

This method is used when you wish to recruit people who are willing to take part and you are not seeking to make claims that these people represent the broader population. Their views may still be important because of their specific experiences (e.g. people with a particular cancer or treatment experience). To recruit this type of sample you could use local media to announce that you are looking for volunteers to take part in a study.

Snowball sampling is one particular type of self-selected sample in which a person who volunteers to participate is asked to suggest other people who might be interested, and so on.

---

*Power calculation means the calculation of a sample size to ensure that statistical judgements are accurate and reliable. See www.statsoft.com/textbook/stpowan.html.
[†]Statistically significant means that it can be demonstrated that the probability of obtaining a result by chance only is relatively low.

Convenience or pragmatic sample

This is a common approach to user involvement exercises. A convenience sample of users is based on those who are easily approached. For example, a questionnaire may be handed out to all patients who attend a clinic on a given day. Information is collected about the characteristics of those who participate, allowing a comparison with those who do not.

When time and resources are limited, a convenience sample provides a snapshot of how people feel about a certain issue at a certain time. This is one of the least costly approaches to user involvement.

Purposive or typical case sampling

This approach is based on identifying a specific category of user or a particular clinic or organisation that you are seeking to approach. You might want to study a setting that was 'typical'. This approach can be useful when you are trying to conduct a case study (e.g. a study of a breast cancer clinic).

Quota (or stratified) sample

A stratified sample is one in which individual participants have to meet some predetermined set of general requirements. These requirements might include age, gender and type of cancer. This approach is typically used by market researchers who look for a certain number of respondents in each of several categories (age, gender, social class) and then put together the results in a way that matches the population. This approach can be helpful when you want to conduct a focus group and you need to capture the views of a wider audience. It can also be useful when you try to compare two groups that are not equally present in the population.

Probability sample

A probability sample can give a balance between accuracy and cost. This approach is based on each possible respondent having the same probability of being selected to participate. For example, you may need to conduct a survey of 100 prostate cancer patients in your NHS trust. You would need to get a list of all of the patients in your clinic (say there are 1000) and then choose every tenth name, or you could construct a more random sample using a computer program to generate 100 random numbers between 1 and 1000. In each case, any given name on the list has the same 10% chance of being identified.

Example: interviewing people about their experience of user involvement

One of the objectives of the ASWCS study was to develop a questionnaire about users' satisfaction with their involvement.

In order to identify the key issues for this questionnaire, we interviewed users of cancer services who were recruited by means of purposive sampling techniques. We displayed posters in health centres and cancer clinics, issued a press release and added information to the project website.

Using the analysis of the interviews, we developed a questionnaire about satisfaction with user involvement.

Summary checklist

Key points to consider when identifying service users include the following.

- Develop a clear rationale for including particular user and stakeholder groups.
- Include a diverse range of views.
- Consider different recruitment methods (e.g. use of local media, work with voluntary organisations).
- Consider the training and support needs of involved users.
- Make resources available.
- Make all written information clear and accessible.
- Use appropriate sampling methods.
- Consider how the results of any exercise will be fed back to users.

Frequently asked questions

Q: Are health professionals users? Are GPs users?

A: The aims of a user involvement exercise define the type of people that need to be involved. Therefore you could consider healthcare professionals as users of cancer services (e.g. as possible future consumers of health services). The boundaries between patient/carer and health professional may be blurred if a health professional experiences cancer as a user. Their perspective is unique, but in order to avoid tokenism you should include users from different professional backgrounds.

Q: What is the minimum number of user representatives that you should include on a committee?

A: It has been suggested that there should be at least two service users on a committee for two reasons. First, two people can provide support to each other, and second, there will not be grounds for suggesting that the views of service users are unrepresentative. In larger groups, such as a user involvement group, an even split between service users and health professionals is considered ideal.

Q: Can a health professional act as an advocate for service users?

A: An advocate can act as a spokesperson for someone who may be intimidated or have difficulty in articulating their views; a health professional could act as an advocate in these cases. For example, people from ethnic minorities who do not speak English may find it easier to become involved through an advocate.

Q: What about confidentiality?

A: The policy of your organisation on confidentiality should be clear to all of those involved in a user involvement initiative. You should also make it clear to all users that their involvement and their views will not affect the level of the care that they receive.

Q: Are there issues in which users should not be involved?

A: Our experience has shown that there are few issues in which users do not want to be involved. It is normally healthcare professionals who worry about users being too frail or not having the knowledge and skills to get involved. What is important is to offer training and support to ensure that the contribution of patients and carers will make a difference.

Q: What type of support might involved users need?

A: There are several types of support that service users could need. Users should be offered reimbursement for expenses incurred while they are involved (e.g. travel, parking costs, childcare), and in cases where there is a substantial amount of work involved, a honorarium should be provided. For user representatives on a steering group, a project worker offering pre- and post-meeting support is crucial. In some cases psychological support may also be needed.

References

- Department of Health (1995) *Improving the Quality of Cancer Services: a Report by the Expert Advisory Group on Cancer to the Chief Medical Officers of England and Wales*. HMSO, London.

Further reading

- Consumers in NHS Research Support Unit (2002) *A Guide to Paying Consumers Actively Involved in Research.* Consumers in NHS Research Support Unit, London.

A practical guide about the payment of consumers who become actively involved in health and social care research as partners in different stages of the research cycle.

- National Consumer Council (2002) *Consumer Representation: making it work.* National Consumer Council, London.

The National Consumer Council guide lists 14 good practice points for supporting and getting the best out of consumer representatives. Although it is not health specific, its principles are applicable to getting users involved in cancer services.

- Maisel R and Persell Hodges C (1996) *How Sampling Works*. Pine Forge Press, Thousand Oaks, CA.

Defining the aims of user involvement

This section focuses on the *(re)defining the aims of user involvement* stage of the cycle of user involvement.

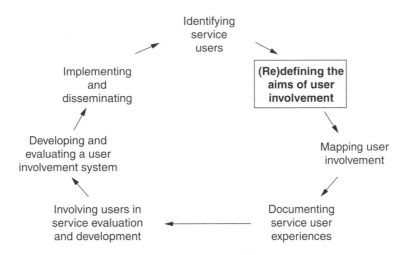

Cycle of user involvement.

In this section, we discuss:

- what 'consensus development' means and some key concerns and issues
- why it is useful
- consensus development methods and their advantages and disadvantages
- the *nominal group technique* consensus development method – what it is, when to use it, its advantages and disadvantages, how to use it and resources required
- the *Delphi technique* consensus development method – what it is, when to use it, its advantages and disadvantages, how to use it and resources required
- frequently asked questions.

Summary of key issues

- User involvement can mean different things to different people. Before starting any user involvement process, it is important to be clear about its aims. At one level, user involvement may be about involving individuals in decisions that affect them (e.g. informing patients about treatment options so that they can make real choices). Although this is important, user involvement also extends much further than this (e.g. involving patients, carers and other stakeholders in decisions about service priorities, including management and resources).
- User involvement can seem threatening to health professionals for a number of reasons, and any discussion about the aims of user involvement is likely to reveal concerns. For example, some may feel that users' input should be limited on the grounds that users may lack specialist knowledge about health services, or that their involvement should be limited because they are too vulnerable to cope with the pressures of decision making.
- Achieving agreement about the aims of user involvement may prove difficult because of these complex issues and because of the wide number of stakeholders who are potentially affected.
- We discuss some of the issues that may arise in relation to defining the aims of user involvement. We introduce the notion of consensus development as a potentially useful approach. Formal and informal consensus methods are identified and the advantages and disadvantages of each are discussed. We outline two particular methods that we used as part of the ASWCS project, namely the *nominal group technique (NGT)* and the *Delphi technique*.
- Our project experience suggests that these methods are useful in bringing to light a range of issues, including fears and concerns held by professionals and users about the process of collaboration. As the consensus process developed, it became apparent that these fears were often ungrounded. They tended to disappear once professionals and users gained experience of working together.
- We suggest that once the aims of user involvement are identified, the process of collaboration can be rewarding both for professionals and for users, who strongly appreciate the benefits of shared understanding that user involvement can bring.

Introduction

Although many people would agree that user involvement is a 'good thing', there is a surprising lack of agreement about what precisely user involvement is. Few people would disagree with the principle that individuals should be involved in decisions that affect them directly, although even this level of involvement has not always been the reality for many patients. In fact, user involvement often means more than this. For example, it is also important to involve users in decisions about service development, although there is likely to be a range of views on how far service users should be able to influence decisions about management and resources within health services.

Some professionals fear that users may not have adequate background information to be able to contribute effectively at this strategic level of involvement, or that the process of involvement will unleash demands from users that they feel unable to meet. There is also a possible fear that feedback from users may be negative. Our project experience suggests that these fears are very real, but they are also often unfounded. Once professionals gain more experience of working with service users they realise that there are significant benefits to be gained from including users in service development.

It is worth considering the reasons why users wish to be involved. Although there are many different motivations, altruism can be a key factor. Users often seek improvements in areas that have affected them directly, such as communication with professionals, although many are aware that their feedback may benefit future users rather than themselves. As well as high-lighting the need for improvements in service provision, users may also wish to feed back positive experiences and make a contribution to a service that they value.

It may be impossible to reach complete agreement on all of the complex issues that relate to user involvement. Furthermore, the aims of user involvement may vary depending on what participants are trying to achieve at any one time. Nevertheless, lack of understanding among professionals about users' experiences and perspectives can get in the way of service development. On the other hand, shared understanding and effective collaboration can harness users' experience and knowledge in order to make positive improvements.

Using consensus development methods to define the aims of user involvement

---

Example: using consensus development methods to define the aims of the ASWCS project

The need to define aims often arises early in any user involvement process, and this was the case in the ASWCS project. It was particularly challenging because of the large number of stakeholders involved – many different professional groups and service users from a large geographical area.

A key aim of this project was to define the aims of user involvement in a way that everyone could agree with as a basis for future service development. We decided to use consensus development methods for this purpose.

What is consensus development?

Consensus development is a tool for measuring the extent to which people agree or disagree about an issue. It is particularly useful in the early stages of user involvement, when there may be a lack of agreement about aims and objectives among a wide range of stakeholders.

Consensus development methods are useful because they can:

• help you to resolve disagreement and work towards agreement on a defined issue
• enable different perspectives to be heard and allow opportunities for discussion and debate
• provide an effective way of involving patients and the public in decision making
• bring together different groups and agencies to explore problems, solutions and priorities.

What are consensus development methods?

A number of different consensus methods are available, and these are increasingly being adopted in a variety of health and social care settings.

Consensus methods can be formal or informal. Formal methods include consensus development conferences, structured group discussion, the Delphi method and the nominal group technique (NGT). Informal methods include focus groups, lobbying and unstructured discussions. In our project, we decided to use the NGT and Delphi methods, and we provide an overview of these below. (Further details about these methods are provided in Part 2, Sections 2A and 2B.)

Advantages and disadvantages

Formal methods have advantages over informal methods in that they make explicit the values and beliefs that guide service development. Informal methods make it difficult to identify who contributes to decisions. Formal methods, on the other hand, allow a wide range of people to contribute, regardless of their status or background. Formal methods can also help the group decision-making process. For example, when formal methods are used, it is hard for very vocal or powerful individuals to dominate the group. These advantages mean that decisions that are reached using formal methods are more likely to receive higher levels of support from participants than those made informally.

One disadvantage of consensus methods concerns the type of definitions reached. For example, everyone might agree with some statements but, like 'motherhood and apple pie', these may be too bland to be really helpful.

It is also worth bearing in mind that the outcomes of consensus development are only as good as the inputs. If participants are not well informed about the issues being discussed, the results will be of limited value. Consensus development should not therefore be seen as providing the final answer. Circumstances may change and there may be a need to revisit debates and issues.

Nevertheless, consensus development can be useful at the stage of defining the aims and scope of user involvement. User involvement is much more likely to be successful if those participating themselves have a chance to be involved in this process and to 'own' the results.

Methods of consensus development: the nominal group technique and the Delphi technique

Anyone can use consensus methods, but our discussion has shown that they need to be used sensitively and with care – whichever method is chosen, defined procedures must be followed. More information about these techniques is available in the Further Reading list at the end of this section. What follows now is an introduction to two of the methods, namely the *nominal group technique (NGT)* and the *Delphi technique*, and an illustration of how these might be used in the process of consensus development in cancer services.

The nominal group technique (NGT)

What it is

The NGT was developed in the USA during the late 1960s (Delbeq *et al.*, 1975). It involves structured group discussion in which selected participants are given an equal chance to participate as well as to influence the outcome. The NGT can produce a number of outcomes that might be useful to policy makers and practitioners. These include single and multiple statements, with levels of agreement or priority indicated by a numerical score.

The NGT can be used in a number of ways, including the following:

- in clinical settings, to aid judgements about whether and how interventions should be carried out
- in policy and service development to aid decisions
- as a tool for education and training.

When to use it

Consensus development can take place at any point during the user involvement cycle, depending on the question being asked and the participants being consulted. The most useful time to use the NGT in consensus development might be during the early stages of the cycle, when you are defining aims and objectives.

The NGT is a useful technique when you need to consult or develop consensus about a key question. It is also useful when it is possible to include participants in a small group discussion. The NGT usually involves a relatively small number of participants, although it is crucial to select participants carefully in order to include relevant interests and perspectives.

The NGT is not useful for exploring multiple questions, as groups would find it difficult to discuss these within the structured approach. It is also less useful when there is a need to consult a large group of people at the same time, although multiple groups can be organised and the results fed back to the larger group in a follow-up exercise (such as the Delphi technique; see below).

You can use the NGT with groups of people from mixed backgrounds as well as from similar backgrounds. Groups from mixed backgrounds may find it more difficult to reach a consensus, but they are also more likely to generate a broader range of issues for consideration. The NGT can be used with participants from a wide variety of backgrounds and it is a relatively democratic technique – it offers everyone who takes part an equal chance to contribute to the discussion and influence the results, and it prevents vocal or powerful individuals from dominating the group.

The NGT can also offer an efficient way of generating information using relatively few resources. However, it does carry the risk of reducing or oversimplifying complex information and disagreements. It may give more weight to majority opinions, and care should be taken if there is a need to include minority views.

Finally, care is needed to make the technique accessible to everyone. For example, you may need to adapt the technique to include people who cannot read or write, people with communication impairments or people who do not share a common language.

Summary of the advantages and disadvantages of the nominal group technique

Advantages
- Useful for exploring a single question
- Useful way of structuring small group discussion
- Can include people from a range of backgrounds
- Draws on a wide range of expertise
- Democratic

Disadvantages
- Difficult to explore more than one question
- Difficult to include large numbers
- Participants must be able to wide read and write
- Outcomes are limited by quality of input
- Minority views can get lost

How to use it

The following outline summarises the main stages in the process, and highlights some key issues that might arise at each stage (*see* Part 2, Section 2A, for a fuller description of this procedure). It is advisable to undertake further reading before carrying out a consensus development exercise using the NGT.

The nominal group technique: summary of procedure

1 Define the question	Identify a single question or statement for discussion
2 Identify the participants	Who will you invite to take part? Try to ensure that all relevant groups are included. Consider social and demographic characteristics as well as those relating to the experience of cancer and the organisation of cancer services
3 Send out information	Identify relevant research or policy documents and give these to participants in advance. Ask them to reflect on the question and make personal notes
4 Run the group	Silent generation of ideas; 'round-robin' reporting; group discussion and scoring
5 Evaluate	Process and outcomes evaluation are needed. Use both qualitative and quantitative methods*

Resources you need: checklist for the nominal group technique

Equipment/resource	*Tasks and things to consider*
Room	Size, comfort, access
Refreshments	Special diets
Background information	Send to participants in advance
Notepaper and pens	
Flipchart and paper or board and markers	
Participants' score sheets	See example in Part 2, Section 3B
Facilitators' score sheets	See example in Part 2, Section 3B
Calculator	
Facilitators	Two facilitators may be needed
	Internal or external?
	Is training required?
Observer	Can contribute to the process, depending on the aims. Is training required?
Administrative support	Invitation letters, feedback of results, etc.

Qualitative data are in the form of words and need different methods of analysis to *quantitative* data, which are in the form of numbers.

Example: consensus development in the ASWCS project using the nominal group technique

This is an example of NGT results in the form of the top ten statements, showing their scoring and rankings based on a session with seven participants.

In this study the initial question was as follows.

What are the key issues to consider when involving cancer service users in service development?

This illustrates the type of statements that may be generated during an NGT session. In this example, the statements were generated by a group of researchers. We show them in the order of final ranking, based on the mean score for each statement. We also show the initial scores given by individuals.

This example illustrates the benefit of a second scoring round, in that some individuals changed their priorities after discussion and reflection on the initial results, and this influenced the final outcome.

Top ten statements

Final ranking	*Statement*	*Initial score (mean, based on rankings out of 10)*	*Individual scores at second round (out of 100)*	*Final score (out of 700)*
1	The need to recognise the different levels of power and control involved, and how far professionals are prepared to go	42 (1st)	100,98,98,90 90,85,70	631
2	The 'ladder of participation' – need to understand how to apply this (i.e. what is appropriate/possible in different instances, not seeing user involvement as a one-off process)	28 (2nd)	100,99,96,95, 95,90,40	615
3	The reality of participation – needs to be on real/equal terms, not lip service	18 (8th)	94,92,92,91, 85,80,60	594
4	Developing a culture of user involvement	26 (4th)	100,100,100, 98,96,50,50	594

continued overleaf

Top ten statements

Final ranking	Statement	Initial score (mean, based on rankings out of 10)	Individual scores at second round (out of 100)	Final score (out of 700)
5	A range of spaces and methods should be provided to listen to people. Is it about individual care or service development?	28 (2nd)	98,97,80,80, 75,75,70	575
6	The need to clarify different forms of user involvement and define these	18 (8th)	100,95,94,90, 82,71,35	567
7	Why involve people? Is it about clinical effectiveness or a moral right?	22 (5th)	99,95,90,75, 70,60,50	539
8	Motivation, vulnerability, stage – people's experience of cancer	22 (5th)	95,90,86,81, 60,60,45	517
9	The need for training for all stakeholders to ensure the effectiveness of their involvement	17 (10th)	93,91,90,72, 70,51,20	487
10	Are we considering users as representatives or representative?	23 (7th)	90,80,75,70, 51,10,5	381

The Delphi technique

What it is

The Delphi technique originated in the late 1940s as a method of aggregating the judgements of a number of individuals in order to improve the quality of decision making (Delbeq *et al.*, 1975). It involves sending questionnaires to participants in a two-stage process, asking them to state to what extent they agree with a series of statements.

The Delphi technique can produce useful consensus statements that can guide policy and service development, for decision making and setting priorities in healthcare. It can be used on its own or with the NGT.

It can allow a wide range of people to contribute to debates and decisions, and has the advantage that participants do not have to meet. This can be useful when there is a need for anonymity, or when groups might be antagonistic towards each other. (An example of a consensus statement produced using the Delphi technique in conjunction with the NGT is provided in Part 2, Sections 3C and 3D.)

When to use it

Like the NGT, the Delphi technique is useful at the beginning of the user involvement cycle, when aims and objectives are being defined.

Unlike the NGT, the Delphi technique can be used to explore a number of different questions. It is especially useful if there is a need for anonymity or it is not possible or desirable for participants to meet. It can be used with groups of people from mixed backgrounds as well as those from similar backgrounds, although participants do need to be able to read and write. The Delphi technique is democratic in that it allows all participants an equal chance of influencing the results although, like questionnaire surveys in general, a lack of response from certain groups can bias the findings towards those who do respond.

The Delphi technique is a quantitative tool and relies on some knowledge of data analysis and statistics. There are many different ways of interpreting the results and different definitions of consensus that can affect the outcomes. For example, if a high threshold of consensus is adopted, the resulting consensus statements may be too bland to be useful. On the other hand, if a low threshold of consensus is adopted, the statements may mask important disagreements. The Delphi technique is of limited use when there is a need to generate rich data or explore subtle disagreements between groups.

Summary of the advantages and disadvantages of the Delphi technique

Advantages
- Can explore a range of questions
- Easy to include large numbers
- Can include people from a wide range of backgrounds
- Draws on a wide range of expertise
- Democratic

Disadvantages
- Needs relatively simple statements
- Participants do not meet so does not allow discussion
- Participants must be able to read and write
- Outcomes limited by quality of input
- Minority views can get lost

How to use it

The following outline summarises the main stages in the Delphi technique process (*see* Part 2, Section 2B for a more detailed description).

The Delphi technique: summary of procedure

1 Preparation	Select main question or prompt. Define potential respondent groups and constituencies. Establish aims, objectives and desired outcomes
2 Identify the participants	Identify all relevant professionals as well as voluntary sector and user groups. Recruit service users through flyers, leaflets, outreach and local media
3 Send out first questionnaire	Generate a list of statements for participants to rate in terms of agreement/disagreement. Send out with covering letter and follow up with reminders
4 Analyse first questionnaire	Calculate mean scores for each statement
5 Send out second questionnaire	Feed back results of the first questionnaire and allow participants to re-rank items in relation to the group judgement
6 Analyse second questionnaire	Calculate final rankings for each statement and decide on your consensus threshold*
7 Create outcomes	You should end up with a consensus statement!
8 Disseminate and evaluate	Use workshops and training sessions to discuss implementation of the consensus statement. Consider publication in professional and academic journals

---

*The level of agreement that will indicate that a consensus has been reached.

Resources you need: checklist for the Delphi technique

Equipment/resource	*Tasks and things to consider*
Background information	Send to participants in advance
Questionnaire design	Need to make sure that this is clear and demonstrates validity. Can use NGT to develop questionnaire
	Allow sufficient time/resources for design and printing
Organiser	Internal or external?
	Is training required?
Statistical support	Drawing up sample and analysing results
Administrative support	Invitation letters, questionnaire distribution, feedback of results, etc.
Background information	
Questionnaire design	

Frequently asked questions

Q: Do I need ethical approval to carry out consensus development?

A: You may need ethical approval if you are using the NGT, Delphi technique or some other technique as part of a research project that involves service users or NHS staff (*see* Part 1, Section 10 on Ethical Issues).

Q: What if a consensus cannot be reached about a particular issue?

A: No one perspective is 'correct' – this depends on the particular context of the service or programme. Although consensus methods do not provide definitive or binding answers, they can help to involve people in defining the aims and scope of user involvement.

Q: Who can use consensus methods?

A: Anyone can use consensus methods, provided that they follow defined procedures. The Delphi technique is a questionnaire survey and relies on some knowledge of statistical data collection and analysis (*see* Further reading list at the end of this section for more information and a list of resources).

Q: Do minority viewpoints get ignored as a result of the consensus development process?

A: Techniques like the NGT and the Delphi technique can give equal weight to majority opinions, depending on the scoring and rating procedures that are used. However, a record of individual votes is always kept, and this allows minority viewpoints to be clearly identified. These may be just as important to policy makers as majority views.

Q: How should consensus be defined?

A: There is no one method for defining consensus. The threshold of consensus can be low or high, depending on the aims of the particular exercise. High thresholds will result in the inclusion of fewer statements than lower thresholds. If unanimity is required, the process may generate no statements at all! There is a need to balance the goal of consensus with that of generating meaningful information.

References

- Delbecq AL, Van de Ven AH *et al.* (1975) *Group Techniques for Program Planning. A guide to nominal group and Delphi processes.* Sage, Thousand Oaks, CA.

Further reading

- Delbecq AL, Van de Ven AH *et al.* (1975) *Group Techniques for Program Planning. A guide to nominal group and Delphi processes.* Sage, Thousand Oaks, CA.

An overview and guidelines for consensus development.

- Black N, Murphy M *et al.* (1999) Consensus development methods: a review of best practice in creating clinical guidelines. *J Health Services Res Policy.* **4**: 236–48.
- Murphy MK, Black NA *et al.* (1998) Consensus development methods and their use in clinical guideline development. *Health Technology Assessment.* **2**(3).

Both of the above provide a critical discussion of consensus methods.

- Redman S, Carrick S *et al.* (1997) Consulting about priorities for the NHMRC National Breast Cancer Centre: how good is the nominal group technique? *Aust NZ J Public Health.* **21**: 250–6.

An example of an application of the NGT in cancer care.

The following provide examples of consensus development using the NGT and the Delphi technique in a variety of healthcare settings:

- Carney O, McIntosh J *et al*. (1996) The use of the Nominal Group Technique in research with community nurses. *J Adv Nurs.* **23**: 1024–9.

- Gallagher M, Hares T *et al*. (1993) The nominal group technique: a research tool for general practice? *Fam Pract.* **10**: 76–81.

- Laufman L, Lammarino NK *et al*. (1981) The nominal group technique: a health education strategy. *Health Educ.* **12**: 17–19.

- Trickey H, Harvey I *et al*. (1998) Formal consensus and consultation: a qualitative method for development of a guideline for dementia. *Qual Health Care.* **7**: 192–9.

SECTION 4

Mapping user involvement

This section focuses on the *mapping user involvement* stage of the cycle of user involvement.

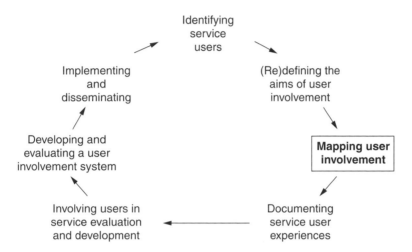

Cycle of user involvement.

In this section, we discuss:

- why you need to find out about current and previous user involvement
- the range of methods you can use to map user involvement activities
- using a mapping questionnaire to collect information from a large group of people – its advantages and disadvantages, when to use it, how to use it and what resources you need
- a case study of an ASWCS mapping exercise, including the key findings
- frequently asked questions about mapping questionnaires.

Summary of key issues

- This section suggests how and why you might find out what user involvement has already taken place. This might be within your own organisation or beyond it.
- We introduce the concept of 'assisted wheel reinvention' to describe the process of learning from what has already taken place when developing new forms of user involvement.
- There are many possible methods of mapping user involvement, which can highlight aspects of services that have not been looked at before. They can also provide a ready resource of knowledgeable and helpful people who know the successes and pitfalls of undertaking user involvement activities.
- The choice of mapping method depends on a number of factors, including the size of the organisation, the number of people undertaking user involvement and the resources available for the exercise. Methods range from evaluating written documents to interviews and meetings with key people.
- If an extensive mapping exercise is needed, a questionnaire survey may be the most appropriate method. We describe the process of undertaking a mapping exercise using a questionnaire designed for this purpose. We discuss the benefits and pitfalls of this approach and include a detailed case study of an ASWCS mapping exercise. The findings of this exercise illustrate the type of information that might be revealed by a mapping exercise, highlighting priorities, opportunities and challenges for service development.

Introduction

Mapping present and previous user involvement

We have already seen how user involvement requires clear, agreed aims. Equally, in order to lead to change, it should take account of the particular needs and history of the organisation undertaking it. This section explores how and why you might find out what user involvement has already taken place in your organisation. This can be useful because it:

- shows what works well in the area
- identifies which service aspects have been looked at before
- provides a ready resource of knowledgeable and helpful people who know the successes and pitfalls of undertaking user involvement activities.

Assisted wheel reinvention

There is no need to repeat work that has been done before – we do not want to reinvent the wheel. For example, before developing questionnaires on patients' and carers' experiences, check whether there are designed and validated questionnaires already available.

One useful way to think about this is in terms of *assisted wheel reinvention*. 'This means catching, learning about successes and spreading new ideas so that local teams can adapt the basic principles for the local situation' (Department of Health, 2001: 10–11).*

If you are seeking to develop and improve user involvement in your organisation, it might not be necessary to start from scratch. Instead, you can use the ideas and experiences that others have had and adapt them to fit in with your particular objectives. However, to do this you need to get an idea of what other people have been doing, the processes they have used and some of the difficulties they have faced.

Finding out about current user involvement

Who do you need to get in touch with to find out more about experiences of user involvement? Who is already doing it? Once you have an idea of who to contact, you need to think about what questions to ask in order to understand how they are undertaking user involvement and what implications and outcomes it has had.

It might be worthwhile considering user involvement that involves voluntary organisations. Often local support groups and cancer charities play an important part in user involvement and can be a source of specialised knowledge and experience.

Methods of mapping user involvement activities

There are a number of methods of mapping user involvement activities within one or more organisations.

- You can *examine documents* such as reports and minutes of meetings.
- You can *talk to groups and individuals* with a dedicated role in this area.
- If the group of people who might be undertaking user involvement activities is relatively small or differs greatly in terms of their roles, responsibilities or work settings, a number of techniques might be suitable, including *meetings or workshops* (*see* Part 1, Section 6).
- If you are seeking to gain information from a large number of people, the most comprehensive approach is to carry out a *survey* using a specially designed mapping questionnaire. This was the approach taken by the ASWCS project, and we describe it in more detail below.

---

*Department of Health (2001) *The NHS Modernisation Board's Annual Report 2000–2001. The NHS Plan: A Progress Report*. Department of Health, London.

The mapping questionnaire

One of the best and least expensive ways of collecting comprehensive information from a large group of people in a standard form is to use a questionnaire.

A mapping questionnaire is a particular type of survey instrument that you can use to:

- document the experiences of different people in an organisation who are undertaking user involvement
- establish what work has been done on user involvement in your organisation
- build up a network of practical expertise about user involvement
- help to identify what has worked and what has been less successful, allowing you to undertake your user involvement using an assisted wheel reinvention model, rather than starting from scratch.

Using a standard mapping questionnaire also means that you can repeat the exercise later, to provide evidence of change over time. It also means that, so long as you have thought about your sample carefully (*see* Part 1, Section 2), your findings will be generalisable* and can tell you about a much larger group of people than those from whom you actually collected information.

Summary of the advantages and disadvantages of the mapping questionnaire

Advantages
- You can collect large amounts of information within a short period of time
- Relatively inexpensive way of collecting a lot of information from a large group of people in a standard way
- Can enable comparisons between different types of respondents or organisations
- Can provide a baseline measurement and, if repeated, demonstrate changes over time

Disadvantages
- Not appropriate if there are only a few people from whom you want to collect information
- Less useful if the people from whom you are collecting information are very diverse
- If there is a limited response, or certain types of organisations or respondents do not respond, the information may not be adequate
- Skill and experience are required to write a good questionnaire and analyse the results

---

*Generalisable findings are those that apply to a population, not just the research sample being studied.

When should you use a mapping questionnaire?

It is important that you map user involvement quite early in the user involvement cycle, before you have formulated your user involvement system. However, as we have already suggested, this initial measurement can be used as a baseline; you can monitor changes and improvements if you repeat the mapping questionnaire at a later date.

How should you devise and use a mapping questionnaire?

You need to go through a number of steps to ensure that your mapping exercise will achieve what you want. In order to establish a baseline measure of user involvement, you need to be sure that:

- the questionnaire is constructed properly
- it is sent to the right people
- it generates sufficient responses
- it is analysed appropriately.

We have set out a summary of the procedure below (for a more detailed description and a sample mapping questionnaire, *see* Part 2, Sections 2C and 3A).

The mapping questionnaire: summary of procedure

1 Identify the participants	Identify the people in your organisation who know, or should know, about user involvement
2 Draft the questionnaire	Think about what information you want to gather. Consider asking some questions that need a short written answer
3 Test the questionnaire	Give your questionnaire to some people who are not in your sample but who should be able to complete it. Use their feedback to improve the wording and design
4 Send out the final questionnaire	Send out the questionnaire to your respondents. Include a covering letter explaining what it is for and a deadline for sending it back to you
5 Send out reminders	Keep good records of who you have sent your questionnaire to and who has returned it. Consider sending one or two reminders

continued overleaf

| 6 Analyse the data | Think about how you can understand the responses. Consider different types of analysis (statistical or content analysis*) |
| 7 Disseminate and evaluate | What was the experience like for the respondents? Did you collect the information you needed? Remember to tell people about what you did and found |

Resources you need: checklist for a mapping questionnaire

Equipment/resource	*Tasks and things to consider*
Finance	Printing and mailing costs
Questionnaire	Design and analysis
Personal computer	
Administrator	Sending out questionnaire and reminders
Co-ordinator	Keeping track of who has responded
	Overall responsibility; overseeing evaluation and interpreting analysis

---

Case study: the mapping exercise in ASWCS

Aims

The aims of the mapping exercise carried out in ASWCS in 2000 were as follows:

- to document the range of definitions of user involvement
- to identify the methods used to involve users
- to identify examples of user involvement within the NHS and other statutory-sector organisations
- to explore how user involvement was understood in relation to cancer services
- to map the variations between different types of organisations across the three health authorities (Avon, Somerset and Wiltshire).

Questionnaire design

In order to design the mapping questionnaire, we reviewed the literature on user involvement and cancer services. We identified the following key aspects of user involvement, which were incorporated into the design of the questionnaire:

- types of user involved
- aim and objectives of user involvement

continued opposite

---

*Content analysis is a method of analysing written data to identify themes, ideas, etc. and the relationship between them.

- level of involvement
- process of selecting/recruiting users
- methods of involvement
- duration of involvement
- outcomes of involvement
- organisational support provided to staff and users.

Pilot study

Before carrying out the main survey we piloted the questionnaire with organisations in a different area that were similar to the ones we wished to study.

(In Part 2, Section 3A we have included the questionnaire that was sent to voluntary organisations and support groups. It may be worth looking at this as well as considering the example below.)

The sample for the statutory sector questionnaire

We sent questionnaires to the following:

- Six Cancer Leads or Public Involvement Leads in the three health authorities
- Five Community Health Council Chief Officers
- Six Directors of Social Services in local councils
- Sixteen Trust Chief Executives, Cancer Managers, Public Involvement Leads or Clinical Governance Directors
- Five Trust Research and Development Co-ordinators
- Twenty-one Primary Care Group Chairs
- Six Hospice Chief Executives or General Managers*
- Six others.[†]

Evaluating responses

In total, we received 40 responses from 71 individuals. Several of the questionnaires were joint responses. Therefore the data include the views of 48 individuals giving an overall response rate of 67.6%. (It is usual to expect a response rate of 40–45% with a questionnaire mailed to people you have not contacted before, when you also send one reminder letter.)

continued overleaf

---

*We accept that hospices are not necessarily part of the statutory sector, as most of them are charities and receive only a minority of their funding from the NHS. However, there is considerable overlap in staffing and close working relationships with NHS trust staff. Furthermore, hospices are directly involved in patient care and structurally are far more similar to statutory organisations than to voluntary sector organisations. This meant that many of the questions we asked statutory sector organisations were relevant to hospices.

[†]We identified individuals using the cancer network's database. The questionnaire also asked respondents to suggest additional individuals who it might be appropriate to contact. These suggestions generated an additional sample of six individuals.

Simply looking at the proportion of people who responded does not tell you whether the answers are biased in any way. It is important to look for patterns among those who do not respond. In this survey, the lowest response rates were among primary care groups – only 10 out of 21 individuals from this group responded. Responses were also relatively low among community health councils – 3 out of 6 individuals from this group responded. However, even for these groups we received responses from at least half the sample.

Overall, we concluded that the responses we received did reasonably represent the views of the statutory sector of cancer service organisations in Avon, Somerset and Wiltshire.

Key findings from the ASWCS mapping exercise
Here we briefly summarise the findings from the ASWCS mapping exercise to illustrate the type of information that such an exercise can reveal, focusing on five key areas.

The findings give a clear picture of what user involvement was going on at the time of the survey in March 2001, as well as highlighting priorities, opportunities and challenges for future service development.

Definitions of user involvement
- The survey found many different definitions of *user* and *user involvement* among people who took part. This lack of consensus may have been a reason why some people did not respond to the questionnaire.
- This lack of consensus also affected the understanding and experience of user involvement. There were huge variations in the amount of user involvement in the different organisations. These differences existed even between NHS trusts within the same health authority.
- Local councils seemed to have greater experience of user involvement than other organisations, such as health authorities. For example, councils were more likely than other organisations to have written policies and the appropriate infrastructure to support user involvement activities. User involvement was generally seen as part of the organisational culture of the responding councils, and a key mechanism for empowering users.
- The survey demonstrated that the vast majority of people who took part supported the principle of user involvement. This was the case in both the voluntary and statutory sectors. Furthermore, there was a clear consensus that users should be involved in both the evaluation and development of cancer services. However, there was a lack of experience, knowledge and supportive infrastructure with regard to how to involve users in practice.

Policies for user involvement
- The survey showed that few written policies on user involvement existed and that staff knowledge of such policies tended to be poor.

continued opposite

- There was some evidence of plans to develop policies, and many people acknowledged that such policies needed to be developed.

User involvement in primary care
- User involvement had a relatively low profile within primary care groups.
- Primary care group respondents seemed to be the least aware of policies or practices with regard to this issue, although a number of these respondents suggested that approaches to user involvement were currently being developed.

Methods for involving users
- There was evidence of both direct and indirect involvement. (Indirect involvement takes place when users contribute information to decision making, while direct involvement takes place when users are enabled to actually take part in decision making; *see* Part 1, Section 1.)
- Many of the examples of user involvement that we found took the form of information gathering. There was a significant overlap between research methods and methods for involving users. This suggests that much of what is called 'user involvement' actually involves collecting data from users, as part of research projects or accreditation exercises.
- There was significant evidence of users serving as representatives on committees. Respondents from the voluntary sector reported that this approach was empowering for those users who took part.

Training and support
- The survey explored the level of training in user involvement that was provided for staff and users in the statutory sector. Limited training seemed to exist, although some ongoing practical support was provided for involved users.

Frequently asked questions on mapping questionnaires

Q: Do I need approval from an Ethics Committee?

A: No, just as with audit processes, most user involvement activities are considered to be part of service and staff development rather than research. If you are considering a more research-oriented type of activity, it may be worthwhile checking with your Research and Development department or talking to the Secretary to the Ethics Committee (*see* Part 1, Section 10).

Q: When is it best to carry out a mapping exercise?

A: It is worth doing a mapping exercise quite early in the process of designing your user involvement system. It will help you to find out who else is doing similar work. The people you identify can be helpful in overcoming some of the problems you may encounter, and they may well be interested in working with you.

Q: How do I identify voluntary organisations?

A: Usually voluntary organisations develop to serve particular types of people. If they are relevant to your clinical area, they may be advertised in a waiting-room. Many NHS trusts now have Patient Information Centres that provide useful information about voluntary organisations. Sometimes local councils provide funding for voluntary organisations, and they may be able to suggest useful contacts.

Q: What is an acceptable response rate?

A: Typically, if you send a postal questionnaire to people you do not know, you obtain a response rate of about 30%. If you send out a second questionnaire and letter, the response rate rises to 40%. However, our experience in healthcare where people know the organisation sending the questionnaire suggests that you are likely to obtain a response rate of 50–70%. It may be worth considering phoning the people you really want to hear from.

Q: How do I analyse the data?

A: If you do not have a background in analysis of questionnaire data, you should probably ask for some help from your Research and Development department. Some of the material may be easy for you to think about, but to do so systematically requires training and experience.

Further reading

- Frazer L (2000) *Questionnaire Design and Administration: a practical guide.* John Wiley & Sons, Brisbane.
- NHS Modernisation Agency (2001) *Supporting Delivery: NHS Modernisation Agency Work Programme 2001/2002.* Department of Health, London.
- Seymour S (1982) *Asking Questions: a practical guide to questionnaire design.* Jossey-Bass, Oxford.

SECTION 5

Documenting service user experiences

This section focuses on the *documenting service user experiences* stage of the cycle of user involvement.

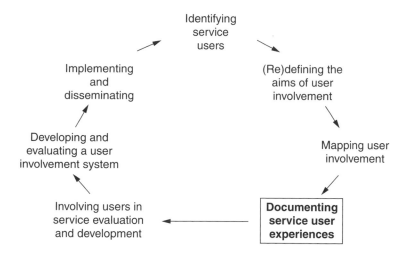

Cycle of user involvement.

In this section, we discuss:

- the concept of the *cancer journey* to describe the stages of medical care that people with cancer experience
- methods of capturing service users' experience
- focus groups – what they are, why and when to use them, their advantages and disadvantages, the resources that are required, how to run them, and a case study of a focus group
- interviews – why and when to use them, the resources that are required, how to conduct them, and a case study of the use of interviews to document user experiences
- frequently asked questions about capturing user experiences.

Summary of key issues

- Examining people's experiences of healthcare services is an important part of the user involvement cycle.
- The different stages of medical care that people with cancer are likely to pass through are sometimes known as the *cancer journey*. These stages include investigation, diagnosis and treatment. Patients experience the cancer journey in different ways, and for some of them, medical procedures are not the most significant markers of their experience of cancer. However, the concept of the cancer journey provides a useful way of thinking about the likely physical, psychological and social impact of cancer for different people at different stages. When collecting information from service users, it is important to be sensitive to all of these factors.
- You can use different methods for collecting information from service users about their experiences. The choice depends on the type of service users involved, the resources available and the type of information that is being sought.
- You can use questionnaires to document users' experiences, especially when relatively straightforward information is being sought from large numbers of people.
- Finding out what patients think about services often raises complex and sensitive issues that are difficult to capture in a questionnaire. Two further methods of collecting information are focus groups and interviews. Both of these might be more useful than questionnaires for sensitive subject matter.
- Focus groups work well if the topic is suitable for a group discussion. You can use them to gather information from groups of people with similar backgrounds, or to explore multiple perspectives with groups composed of people from a range of backgrounds.
- Interviews are the most suitable method for seeking personal or confidential information, or for when you need to provide individual attention and one-to-one support to service users, such as those with communication impairments.
- Using a combination of methods is likely to improve the reliability of any information-gathering exercise, and is more likely than a single method to meet a range of different needs.
- Whatever method is used, it is important to give feedback to participants about any actions or decisions that are taken as a result of the exercise.

Introduction

Patients and carers are the experts in receiving health services, just as health professionals are the experts in providing them. Service users' experiences are an invaluable tool in the process of evaluating and developing services. There are two main aspects of investigating service user experiences. Here we look at ways of capturing the experiences and needs of those receiving services, while in Part 1, Section 6 we focus on involving service users in evaluating the effectiveness of services.

The cancer journey

Before looking at possible methods for documenting service user experience, it is useful to consider the different stages of medical care that people with cancer are likely to pass through. This is sometimes known as the *cancer journey,** and it is summarised in Figure 5.1.

Not all of the different stages of medical care relate to every person with cancer.

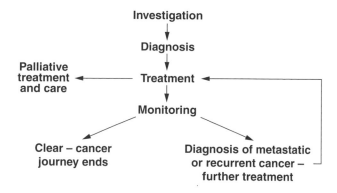

Figure 5.1: The cancer journey.

The first stage is *investigation,* when a person is referred for specific tests to find out whether they have cancer. Following the tests a decision will be made as to whether or not the person actually does have cancer.

---

*National Cancer Alliance (1995) *Directory of Cancer Specialists*. National Cancer Alliance, Oxford.

The second stage is *diagnosis*, when a person is first told that they have cancer. Different types of treatment will be discussed with the patient and a decision made about what to do.

This leads to the *treatment* stage, which can include surgery, radiotherapy, chemotherapy or some combination of these. Treatment often takes place over a period of time and may involve different medical specialists. It can take place in different clinics or even in different hospitals.

After being treated, the person who was diagnosed with cancer is asked to see a medical specialist at regular intervals. At these meetings the doctor will check to see whether there is any evidence that the cancer has returned. This stage of the cancer journey is called *monitoring*, and it can last for a long time.

After five years of regular monitoring, people who were diagnosed with cancer are defined as 'clear' and no longer have cancer. For these people the cancer journey ends here.

If the cancer returns or is found in a different place to that where it was initially diagnosed, the *diagnosis of metastatic or recurrent cancer* is the next stage of the cancer journey. This can lead to another *treatment* stage.

For some people there will be no cure for their cancer, and treatment is about reducing pain or helping them to live longer. This is known as *palliative treatment*. Many people who are being treated for metastatic or recurrent cancer will also receive specialist pain treatment, and sometimes this is called *palliative care*.

Methods of capturing service users' experience

There are a number of ways of investigating the experiences of service users. Written materials, including writings by people with cancer, often provide useful insights, as can creative arts, including theatre and film.

When seeking to collect specific information for a particular programme of service development, the use of a combination of techniques can often improve the range and reliability of the data. Below we look at the following three methods in detail and consider how they might be used:

- focus groups
- interviews
- questionnaires.

When asking service users about their experiences, it is important to be aware of the emotional issues that may be raised and to provide appropriate support.

Focus groups

What are focus groups?

A focus group is an organised discussion with a small group of people using their experiences, feelings and beliefs to focus on a specific topic. The main aim is to encourage discussion of a particular topic among a range of service users, in order to collect information on opinions, beliefs, experiences and attitudes. Groups usually tend to last for between one and two hours.

An important feature of this technique is the interaction between participants. The most crucial role of a facilitator or moderator is to channel the discussion.

Ideally, a group should be repeated several times with different participants, using the same framework of topics.

Why use focus groups?

Focus groups are a good way to collect a large amount of information in a short time. They are interactive and spontaneous, and are a good way to generate in-depth qualitative* data. Focus groups are particularly suitable for discussing sensitive topics, and can be used to explore and develop consensus around an issue.

When might focus groups not be useful?

There are a number of situations where focus groups might not be the best method to use, including the following:

- when you want to obtain information from a large number of people. The best size for a focus group is 6 to 10 people. Although you can hold several groups on the same topic, this is not an efficient way to obtain information from a large number of respondents because it requires a lot of time and other resources
- when you do not have access to specialist resources. You need an experienced facilitator to run a focus group successfully, facilities for recording and transcribing, and sufficient time to analyse qualitative data
- when you want to generalise your findings to a wider group of people. It is almost impossible to obtain a representative sample of people in any focus group. Therefore focus groups are not suitable if you want to make definite statements about a wider population.

---

*Qualitative data are presented in the form of words, in contrast to quantitative data, which are presented in the form of numbers.

Summary of the advantages and disadvantages of focus groups

Advantages
- You can collect large amounts of information in a short period of time
- Generates in-depth qualitative data
- Group discussion promotes the development of ideas and attitudes
- A good way of developing themes and ideas for further research

Disadvantages
- Some people are not comfortable working in groups
- Analysis is complex and time-consuming
- The small numbers involved make it difficult to achieve a representative sample
- It can be difficult to identify themes from multiple viewpoints

When to use focus groups

Focus groups are particularly suited to the early stages of research, when they can be a good way to develop hypotheses and inform the design of questionnaires and interview schedules. You can also use them in the later stages as a way of providing participants with feedback on your findings and evaluating the project from service users' point of view.

Resources you need: checklist for a focus group

Equipment/resource	*Tasks and things to consider*
Room	Size, comfort, access
Refreshments	Special diets
Finance	Expenses of participants
Tape recorder	Sound quality, microphone positioning
Transcribing machine	
Background information	To send to participants
PC	Analysis and report writing
Facilitator	Internal or external?
Co-ordinator	Dissemination activities
Observer	An alternative or back-up to tape recording
Administration	Transcribing, sending out invitations, background materials, etc.

How to run a focus group

Focus groups involve a lot of organisation, so you need to start planning several weeks before you aim to hold a group. We have set out a summary of how to plan a group below (*see* Part 2, Section 2D for a more detailed description).

Running a focus group: summary of procedure

1 Define your aims	Be clear about what you want the focus group(s) to achieve
2 Identify the participants	Who should take part? Try to ensure that all relevant groups are included. Consider social and demographic characteristics as well as those relating to the experience of cancer and the organisation of cancer services
3 Find a facilitator	Effective facilitation is essential to a good focus group. This involves good communication skills and an awareness of group dynamics. Preferably this person should be neutral (i.e. not an employee of your organisation) and, if your budget will allow for it, a professional facilitator is the preferred option
4 Prepare a script	Be clear about what you are going to say to help your group run smoothly
5 Make preparations	Send out invitations with background information on the topic area and focus groups. Book a suitable venue, taking into account comfort, size and access
6 Run the group	Be there early to welcome people as they arrive. Tape record the proceedings and arrange for someone to take notes
7 Analyse the data	Use content analysis to identify themes and interactions
8 Evaluate and disseminate	Look at how it worked and what you found, using both qualitative and quantitative methods. Let people know what you have done and what you found, including the participants

---

Case study of a focus group

ASWCS wanted to investigate service users' experiences of participating in a local user involvement group.

We chose a focus group as the most appropriate method because it would enable a semi-structured discussion involving 8 to 10 participants. All members of the user involvement group were invited, so the potential participants were self-selecting.

continued overleaf

We enlisted an experienced facilitator with expertise in user involvement to run the groups.

We developed a topic guide from a review of previous research in order to provide a *general* structure for the groups. Themes included the following:

- reasons for joining the group
- the meaning of user involvement
- methods of involvement
- how effective involvement is.

Two focus groups were held at the local cancer service offices, with a total of 16 participants. The groups were taped, transcribed and then analysed for content.

The following key themes emerged from the groups.

- The benefits of user involvement include better services, bringing service users and professionals closer together, and increased democracy.
- It is important to make user involvement effective rather than tokenistic.
- Training and support for both service users and health professionals is essential for effective user involvement.
- Successful user involvement requires proper resourcing, including personnel, equipment and money.
- Information and communication are central to effective user involvement.
- Lack of time and professional defensiveness are two of the main barriers to user involvement.
- Different methods of user involvement are appropriate for different people and different purposes.

We disseminated these key findings in several ways, including a project report, conference presentations and peer-reviewed publications.

Interviews

Interviews are a widely used method of collecting information on people's feelings, beliefs and opinions. They can be divided into three main categories.

- *Structured interviews* tend to use fixed questions (e.g. 'Would you describe your health as good, fair or poor?').
- *Semi-structured interviews* are based on more open questions (e.g. 'How would you describe your own health?').
- *Unstructured interviews* deal with broad subject areas (e.g. 'Tell me about your own health experiences').

Each type of interview has advantages and disadvantages. In general, the less structured the interview, the greater the resources required in terms of the time needed to conduct the interview, the level of interviewer skill, and the difficulty of analysis.

Why conduct interviews?

Interviews are a good way of obtaining in-depth information on complex subjects. Their one-to-one nature makes them suitable for dealing with sensitive subjects in a confidential way.

When to conduct interviews

Interviews are often conducted at the beginning of a study in order to identify themes for further investigation. For example, they are a good way to develop the content of a questionnaire.

When might interviews not be useful?

In some instances, interviews might not be useful. For example, they may not be suitable if you want to collect information from a large number of people because they often require a lot of resources, particularly time.

Resources you need: checklist for interviewing

Equipment/resource	*Tasks and things to consider*
Room	Size, comfort, access
Refreshments	Special diets
Finance	Will you pay participants for their expenses and/or time?
Tape recorder	Sound quality, microphone positioning
Interview schedule	How structured should it be?
Transcribing machine	
Background information	To send to participants
PC	For analysis and report writing
Interviewer	Internal or external? Is training required?
Observer	An alternative or back-up to tape recording
Administration	Transcribing, sending out invitations, background materials, etc.

How to conduct interviews

Below is a summary of how to conduct interviews (for a more detailed description of this method, *see* Part 2, Section 2E).

Conducting interviews: summary of procedure

1 Define your aims	Be clear about what you want to find out from your interviews
2 Identify the participants	Who should you interview? Try to ensure that all relevant groups are included. Consider social and demographic characteristics as well as those relating to the experience of cancer and the organisation of cancer services
3 Develop an interview schedule	Identify key themes from the literature and consider pilot interviews. Structured interviews will usually require a greater number of questions
4 Prepare a script	It is important to use the same form of words for all of your interviews
5 Choose venues	Offer participants a choice of venue, including somewhere neutral. Also consider the safety of the interviewers
6 Conduct the interviews	Taping interviews is often the best option. It is important to offer interviewees any support they might need
7 Analyse the data	Use content analysis to identify general themes and specific quotes
8 Evaluate and disseminate	Look at how it worked and what you found, using both qualitative and quantitative methods. Let people know what you have done and what you found, including the participants

Case study of the use of interviews to document service user experiences

As part of a recent study of user involvement in cancer services in Avon, Somerset and Wiltshire, ASWCS conducted interviews with 37 cancer service users.

The main aim was to identify themes with regard to satisfaction with user involvement, which could contribute towards the development of a questionnaire about satisfaction with user involvement.

We recruited participants by placing posters and leaflets in appropriate locations (doctors' surgeries, hospitals, etc. and a local prostate cancer clinic).

continued opposite

We developed a semi-structured interview schedule, based on pilot interviews and a review of the relevant literature. Interviews were taped, transcribed and then analysed for content using computer software.

Dissemination took place in a number of ways, including a final report, peer-reviewed publications, conference presentations and a newsletter.

Content analysis* of the interviews produced a number of key findings.

- Respondents covered a range of cancer types (including breast, prostate, tongue, bone, ovarian, bowel, liver and lung cancer) and treatments (including radiotherapy, chemotherapy, surgery and hormone therapy). In total, there were 19 male and 18 female interviewees, with ages ranging from 39 to 81 years. All but seven interviewees had had some experience of user involvement, including taking part in treatment decisions, questionnaire-based service evaluation/feedback, voluntary sector activities, drug trials, making a complaint and fundraising.
- There appeared to be limited understanding of the concept of 'user involvement'. Many respondents saw it just in terms of taking part in decisions about their own care. Fewer went beyond this to discuss involvement in service evaluation and development in ways such as surveys, treatment trials, support groups, committee membership and fundraising.
- The most common motivation to become involved was to help other people, particularly in terms of taking part in drug trials.
- The main barriers to user involvement were lack of awareness, limited opportunity, unwillingness to take part in groups and professional resistance.
- Information and communication were highlighted as crucial factors in successful user involvement.

Questionnaires

Questionnaires are often used to document service user experiences. They can be completed in a number of ways, including face-to-face, by telephone or through self-completion. You can use questionnaires to collect both quantitative and qualitative data, and they are suited to both open and closed questions.

For more information on the advantages and disadvantages of questionnaires, how to use them, and an example of putting them into practice, *see* Part 1, Section 4 on mapping user involvement.

---

*Content analysis is a method of analysing written data to identify themes, ideas, etc. and the relationships between them.

Frequently asked questions

Q: Should service users be paid for taking part in user involvement activities?

A: Yes. Users are giving up their time and should be paid something. Paying users acknowledges the value of their contribution, and it allows a far broader range of people to participate. It is usual to reimburse participants for any cost incurred in taking part, such as travel and childcare expenses. Check your organisation's policy on user involvement and see the *Consumers in NHS Research* website: www.conres.co.uk

Q: What is the ideal size for a focus group?

A: Usually focus groups should have at least four people in them, as this ensures that there are enough different experiences to enable a good discussion. If there are more than 12 people it is difficult for everyone to have their say, so the ideal number is between 4 and 12 people.

Q: Is the cancer journey universal?

A: Not all people with cancer go through all of the phases of the cancer journey, but it is a useful framework for thinking about the experience of different stages such as being diagnosed, treated for and living with cancer. There are specific differences in the cancer journey relating to cancer type and the particular organisation of cancer services in an area.

Q: Can findings from user involvement activities be generalised?

A: The user experiences you are trying to gather are specific to the individuals involved. Information on the particular issues that were either problematic or went really well can be useful for improving services. However, not all people will respond the same way. Most findings will not hold for everyone, but improving the service is likely to benefit everyone.

Q: What type of support should be provided to involved users?

A: Sometimes asking people about their experiences can be personally upsetting to them. When you are organising a user involvement activity, consider what sources of support you can provide directly and what others you can help the user to access. It is useful to have at least two people undertaking most activities, so that one can be available for helping someone who is upset. Often just going out of the room with them and having a quiet talk and a cup of tea can make a huge difference.

Q: What type of support should be provided to people who organise user involvement activities?

A: Asking people about their experiences of illness can also be upsetting to those who are organising activities. Everyone involved in user involvement projects should be encouraged to consider where they will obtain support if their work is personally upsetting.

Q: Are users' views objective?

A: No one is entirely objective or neutral. Users bring particular knowledge based on their experience, and they can ensure that discussion is relevant to the needs of people at the receiving end of services.

Further reading

- Barbour R and Kitzinger J (1999) *Developing Focus Group Research: politics, theory and practice.* Sage, London.

- Barley V, Daniel R *et al.* (1999) *Meeting the Needs of People with Cancer for Support and Self-Management: summary report.* Bristol Cancer Help Centre, Bristol.

- Bell S, Brada M *et al.* (1996) *'Patient-Centred Cancer Services?': what patients say.* National Cancer Alliance, Oxford.

- Bloor M, Frankland J, Thomas M and Robson K (2001) *Focus Groups in Social Research.* Sage, London.

- Jackson CJ and Furnham A (2000) *Designing and Analysing Questionnaires and Surveys. A manual for health professionals and administrators.* Whurr Publishers Ltd, London.

- Macmillan Cancer Relief (1997) *The Cancer Guide.* Macmillan Cancer Relief, London; www.macmillan.org.uk/cguide/2journey.html

- Newell R (1993) *Interviewing Skills for Nurses and Other Health Care Professionals: a structured approach.* Routledge, London.

SECTION 6

Involving users in service evaluation and development

This section focuses on the *involving users in service evaluation and development* stage of the cycle of user involvement.

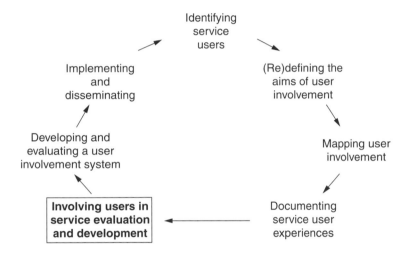

Cycle of user involvement.

In this section, we discuss:

- the importance of involving users in service evaluation and development
- methods of involving users – workshops, questionnaires, focus groups and partnerships forums (user groups)
- workshops in more detail – why and when to run them, their advantages and disadvantages, the resources required, and how to run them
- partnership forums (user groups) in more detail – their functions and issues with regard to setting them up
- examples of two user groups in ASWCS
- frequently asked questions.

Summary of key issues

- Health professionals in a range of disciplines are increasingly aware of the need to evaluate their services. However, in 'evidence-based healthcare' the user's voice is not always heard. This section considers ways of involving users both directly and indirectly in service evaluation and development.
- Although collecting information from service users can be extremely useful, user involvement can go further. Methods are available for enabling users to contribute to decision making about a wide range of service development issues.
- We briefly discuss questionnaires and focus groups in the context of service evaluation and development, and introduce two new methods, namely workshops and partnership forums. Workshops offer a useful method of bringing people from different backgrounds together for problem solving, and can be used at various stages of service development. Partnership forums provide the opportunity to involve users in a more formal, longer-term capacity.
- Partnership forums take a number of different forms. They may consist of mixed groups, including professionals and users, and can include other stakeholders, such as complementary therapists or members of the public. They generally raise the profile of user perspectives within organisations, and they can have formal links with NHS structures as well as acting informally in an advisory capacity.
- We discuss some of the issues that need to be considered when setting up a partnership group. We end with examples, namely the User Involvement Group and the Cancer Forum, both of which are well established within ASWCS.

Introduction

Part 1, Section 5 looked at ways of capturing the experiences and needs of those receiving services. In this section we focus on how to include service users in the evaluation and development of services.

Evaluating service provision

There are many aspects of service provision that we can ask service users to evaluate, including the quality of the service, where it is provided and when it is provided. Asking about gaps in the services can also help service development.

Health professionals in a wide range of disciplines are increasingly encouraged to investigate the impact and effectiveness of their practice. However, in 'evidence-based healthcare'* the user's voice is not always

---

*Healthcare that uses all of the available evidence to identify best practice.

heard. Users have seldom been consulted about the design and implementation of evaluation, and their views about the value of different interventions have not always been sought. This situation is now changing as the principle of patient and public participation is increasingly applied to healthcare evaluation at all levels. Services can be evaluated on an ongoing basis, at regular intervals, or before and after particular changes have been introduced.

Part 1, Section 5 discussed different methods of collecting information from service users for the purposes of service development and evaluation. Finding out what service users think can be extremely valuable, although it is important to give people who have taken part feedback about the outcomes of this indirect form of involvement.

It is also possible to involve users directly in service development and evaluation (*see* Part 1, Section 1). Direct involvement, which occurs when users contribute directly to decision making, can affect a wide range of service development issues. Users can be directly involved in a variety of ways, through membership of committees, advisory groups and lay forums (an overview of methods of user involvement is provided in Part 2, Section 1).

Here we offer examples of methods that have worked well within our own project, including workshops, focus groups, feedback questionnaires and partnership groups.

Methods of involving users in service evaluation

Workshops

Workshops are activity-based groups that provide a hands-on way of defining and solving problems. They require a lot of preparation, and should ideally provide a balance between information provision and participation. As with any user involvement initiative, it is important to consider what support service users may need when they take part.

Why use workshops?

Workshops are an excellent way to involve service users in identifying and solving problems with regard to service delivery.

You can also use them to:

- involve service users in designing patient information
- collate and share information on best practice.

When might workshops not be useful?

Workshops are not an effective way of collecting information from a large number of people. You should think about using a questionnaire for this purpose.

Workshops are suitable for producing definite outcomes. If you want a more general discussion of ideas and experiences with regard to services, a focus group is probably better.

When to use workshops

You can hold workshops at various stages in a project.

- You can use them at the beginning of an evaluation exercise in order to engage individuals and identify problems to be solved.
- Later they can be useful as a way of refining ideas or breaking problems down into smaller parts.
- Towards the end of a user involvement project, they can be a good way to test and refine ideas and materials that you have developed.

Summary of the advantages and disadvantages of workshops

Advantages
- They are a good way to engage people in an evaluation exercise and promote ownership of the outcomes
- They can be a good way to provide feedback to user involvement participants
- Group discussion promotes the development of ideas and attitudes

Disadvantages
- They require a considerable amount of commitment and time on the part of participants
- A lot of preparation is required
- The small numbers involved make it difficult to achieve a representative sample

---

Resources you need: checklist for workshops

Equipment/resource	*Tasks and things to consider*
Room	Size, comfort, access. You may need several rooms if you plan to split up into smaller groups
Refreshments	Special diets
Finance	Will you pay participants for their expenses and/or time?

continued opposite

Evaluation sheet	It is best to use a common format for evaluating different workshop sessions
Background information	To send to participants
Facilitators	Each session needs a facilitator and possibly an assistant
Materials	Flipcharts, pens, paper, etc.
Administration	Booking venue, sending out invitations, background materials, etc.

How to run a workshop

Below is a summary of how you might organise a workshop (*see* Part 2, Section 2H for a more detailed description).

Running a workshop: summary of procedure

1 Define your aims	Be clear about what you want to achieve by running a workshop
2 Identify the participants	Do you want to include staff as well as service users? Send out some background information with the invitations
3 Plan the workshop	Develop a structure and consider breaking the overall theme down into smaller, more manageable tasks
4 Choose a venue	Think about access, comfort and size. You might need several rooms to run smaller sessions
5 Run the workshop	How will you record the proceedings? Ask participants to complete an evaluation form before they leave
6 Analyse the data	Draw together the outcomes of individual sessions
7 Evaluate and disseminate	How did it go and what did you find? How will you put your findings into practice?

Questionnaires

We discussed the use of questionnaires in Part 1, Section 4, but here it is worth making the following points.

• Questionnaires can provide an effective way of involving users in evaluating services.

- You can administer them in a number of ways, including face-to-face interview, telephone interview or self-completion.
- They can include quantitative and qualitative data, and are suited to both open and closed questions.

Questionnaires are particularly useful if you want to obtain the views of a large number of service users. They are also a good way of comparing users' views at different points in time, such as before and after changes in service provision.

When using questionnaires in this way, it is important to think about sampling in order to make sure that the information is as accurate as possible (we discussed sampling methods in detail in Part 1, Section 2).

There are practical issues to consider when drawing up a sample of service users. Take the example of a questionnaire to be posted to a random sample of cancer patients in order to measure their satisfaction with cancer services. Official records are far from infallible, so careful checking of your sample is essential to make sure that you reach the right people. It is especially important to avoid sending questionnaires to people who have not actually had cancer, or who are no longer alive. You should check by inspecting patient records (subject to necessary ethical approval) or through the relevant consultants.

Case study: using a questionnaire to evaluate service user satisfaction

One aim of a Department of Health-funded project was to develop a tool to evaluate service users' satisfaction with their level of involvement in the provision and development of cancer services. This questionnaire also contained a section designed to measure general satisfaction with cancer services.

Respondents were asked to rate a series of 38 statements on a five-point scale ranging from 'Agree Strongly' to 'Disagree Strongly'. The questionnaire was piloted with 60 volunteers who had some experience of user involvement, and will be further tested on a sample of 600 cancer patients.

The full questionnaire can be found in Part 2, Section 3H.

Focus groups

As we discussed in Part 1, Section 5, a focus group is an organised discussion among a small group of people using their experiences, feelings and beliefs to focus on a specific topic. This can be a very effective method of evaluating the views and experiences of service users with regard to a particular service. Focus groups are especially suitable for discussing sensitive topics, and can be used to measure and develop consensus around an issue.

Because the size of a focus group is 6 to 10 people, they are not an effective way to obtain the views of large numbers of service users. Questionnaires are often better for this.

Methods of involving users in service development

We have listed other methods of involving service users directly in the decision-making process in Part 2, Section 1, but we now focus specifically on partnership forums.

Partnership forums (user involvement groups)

Partnership forums (sometimes called user involvement groups) have several key functions.

- They provide a visible presence and role for users in a healthcare setting.
- They demonstrate organisational commitment to gaining a user perspective.
- They provide an ongoing base against which to evaluate and assess service development.
- Depending on how they are constituted, they can contribute directly to service development as well as providing useful information.

Although there are no set rules for user groups, there are some principles that might be helpful. In general, user groups should not be seen as support groups for individuals, but as forums for influencing and monitoring services development.

Issues with regard to setting up partnership forums

There are several key questions you should ask when setting up a partnership forum or user group, including the following.

- Who is the group for? Is it for patients, carers, the general public, voluntary groups, healthcare professionals or complementary therapists?
- How does the group feed into NHS organisations? Is it a subgroup of a committee that is able to influence policy decisions? Or is it a more informal advisory group?
- Where should the group meet? In NHS meeting rooms, on neutral ground, or in the community?
- What are the aims of the group? To be involved in service planning at the outset, to comment on options, or to evaluate changes once they have taken place?
- Who will lead the group? Will it be a partnership between users, the voluntary sector and healthcare professionals, or will one group lead and set the direction?

• When will the group meet? Who will be able to come and who will find it difficult if the group meets in the daytime, in the evening or at the weekend?

You also need to address practical questions, including the following.

• Who will book the venue and refreshments? And who will pay for these?
• Will there be papers? And who will write, copy and circulate these?
• Will users be paid their expenses?
• Will users be paid for their time?

Hopefully, Cancer Partnership Project funding will help to address some of these practical issues. Further work is still required on paying users for their time, although there is increasing recognition of the importance of this issue and the need for clarity.

Finally, user groups need to consider the role and responsibilities of their members.

• Is the group open or closed?
• Who can attend and for how long?
• What qualities, information or experience are members expected to bring?

A full consideration of these issues will help new or existing groups to review their work and establish themselves as robust and sustainable. Addressing these issues will maximise the influence that user groups have on the NHS, and will help to ensure that the development of cancer services is clinically progressive, financially secure and patient centred.

Example: ASWCS user involvement group and cancer forum

ASWCS has two groups that are run in partnership with cancer service users.

User Involvement Group
The first is the User Involvement Group, which is a partnership between patients, carers, voluntary groups and healthcare professionals. The User Involvement Group has a rotating chair, with one user and one healthcare professional co-chairing each meeting. Meetings are generally held over lunch-time, and members are paid their expenses for attendance.

The group focuses on ensuring that patients and carers are fully aware of local developments in cancer services, and that issues of local concern are fed back into the cancer network agenda. The group is well established

continued opposite

within the cancer network and has formal membership of the network Board and Co-ordinating Group. An employee of the cancer network team facilitates the group.

Cancer Forum
The second partnership group in ASWCS is the Cancer Forum. This has its roots in the voluntary sector and healthcare professionals with a lead in education and training. The Cancer Forum has a steering group that consists of patients, carers, voluntary sector members and healthcare professionals.

  The Forum has a more free-thinking role than the User Involvement Group, probably due to its roots in education and training. It serves as an information exchange and an opportunity to broaden horizons. The Forum is funded by the cancer network (with funding from Macmillan Cancer Relief) and is facilitated by an employee of a voluntary sector organisation.

Frequently asked questions

Q: What aspects of services can you ask users to evaluate?

A: Anything of which they have experience, including the quality of services provided, where and when services are provided, or any gaps in service provision which they can identify.

Q: Are some methods better than others for involving users in service evaluation?

A: Questionnaires are a good way of asking a large number of users for basic information on their experiences and opinions, whereas focus groups can provide more detailed information from a smaller number of users.

Q: What should I do with the information that I obtain as a result of involving users in evaluating services?

A: Where possible, it is important to implement the changes suggested by service users. You should also feed the results of any evaluation back to service users (*see* Part 1, Section 8 on implementation and dissemination for details of how to do this).

Q: What is the difference between direct and indirect user involvement?

A: Indirect involvement often involves information gathering by professionals in order to inform service delivery and development, whereas direct involvement means including users in decision making about services (*see* Part 1, Section 1).

Q: How can I include service users in the decision-making process?

A: Partnership forums (sometimes called user involvement groups) are an excellent way of ensuring user input into decisions about services.

Further reading

- Jenkinson C (ed.) (1997) *Assessment and Evaluation of Health and Medical Care: a methods text.* Open University Press, Buckingham.

This textbook provides an overview of different evaluation methods, including the randomised controlled trial (RCT), case–control and cohort studies, systematic reviews, surveys, patient-assessed outcomes, patient satisfaction, qualitative research methods and economic evaluation.

- Shaw IF (1999) *Qualitative Evaluation.* Sage, London.

This text provides a comprehensive introduction to qualitative evaluation methods.

- Gomm R and Davies C (eds) (2000) *Using Evidence in Health and Social Care.* Open University, London.

This text offers a useful overview and discussion of a range of issues associated with using evidence in health and social care practice.

SECTION 7

Developing and evaluating a user involvement system

This section focuses on the *developing and evaluating a user involvement system* stage of the cycle of user involvement.

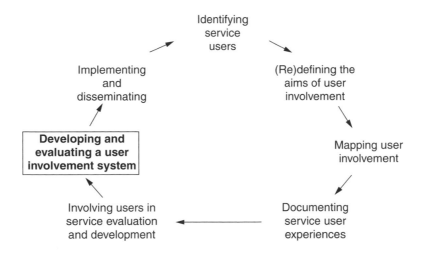

Cycle of user involvement.

In this section, we discuss:

- using the user involvement cycle to develop user involvement systems
- the need for user involvement systems in different organisations and parts of organisations to be co-ordinated and to share information
- national criteria for evaluating user involvement
- criteria developed by ASWCS, and a detailed example of their application in the evaluation of a hospital user involvement programme.

Summary of key issues

- We have emphasised the need to undertake user involvement in a systematic way. In order to achieve this, we have suggested that user involvement should be seen as a continuous cycle rather than a one-off activity. This section discusses the cycle of user involvement in more detail, exploring its different stages.
- Evaluation is a crucial aspect of user involvement. The cycle offers a framework for evaluation as well as development of a systematic user involvement system within organisations. We discuss the evaluation criteria developed by the ASWCS project team. We based these on information provided by service users and professionals in interviews and discussions, as well as drawing on the results of a consensus development exercise within the cancer network.
- Each element of the criteria identifies specific aspects of the user involvement cycle. Together they offer a comprehensive assessment methodology for those seeking to assess how effective user involvement activities are for monitoring and improving services.
- It is helpful to see this type of assessment in terms of process rather than outcomes. User involvement involves complex processes and can never be simply measured. However, the criteria offer a framework for thinking about which aspects of the user involvement system are in place and which need further development. They can either be used as a one-off assessment tool or, more helpfully, as a means of monitoring development over time.

Introduction

So far, we have emphasised the need to undertake user involvement activities in a systematic way. This section discusses the different aspects of a user involvement system and how they fit together. We go on to discuss how user involvement systems can be evaluated, and we present a set of criteria for doing this. We also set out criteria for evaluating a specific user involvement activity.

Our intention is to help you to think through the different aspects of user involvement that are important. This will help to ensure that activities and systems are successful in capturing users' views and applying them as you evaluate and develop your service.

Using the cycle of user involvement

As we have suggested, the idea of a user involvement cycle is one way of helping to ensure a systematic approach to user involvement. The different components of the cycle relate to one another, and each phase of the process (or cycle) builds on and leads to the next phase. The cyclic process helps to ensure that user involvement activities are conducted in a planned way that links directly to changes in service organisation and provision and is continually evaluated by users.

Where does the cycle begin?

If you are beginning to think about setting up a systematic user involvement process, there are a number of different starting points that may be appropriate for you. Most people begin by thinking about the particular aim of the user involvement activity they are considering (*defining aims*). For others, the appropriate starting point relates to a particular category of service users (*identifying service users*). There are no wrong places to begin, but it is important that the different phases of the cycle are all part of the approach you are taking to user involvement.

Consider the example of evaluating activities provided in a day hospice. This initial decision has implications for *identifying service users* whom we want to involve. The most appropriate users are those who can tell you directly about the nature of the service you are examining. In this example, the most appropriate categories of users might be the people who attend the day hospice and their carers. However, it may be that many of the carers do not come to the hospice, and this has implications for rethinking the aim of the user involvement exercise (*defining aims*). There is a close relationship between the aims of the exercise and the categories of service users involved, and we may need to define and redefine these two together.

Once we are clear about the aims of the exercise and the users we want to contact, we need to see whether the type of evaluation we want to undertake has already been done elsewhere (*mapping user involvement*). This process of mapping what has already been done may help us to identify the appropriate method and research tool(s) to adopt in order to *document user experiences* of the day hospice. The particular aim of the example we are looking at is the evaluation of a service, so we need to ensure that the tool(s) we are using are appropriate in that they both document users' experiences and allow us to *evaluate the service*.

When we have collected our data on users' views and experiences and changed the service, we need to examine the approach we have taken. We need to evaluate the user involvement activity we have undertaken and how it fits into a user involvement system (*developing and evaluating a user involvement system*).

Finally, we have to make sure that we feed back our findings and the changes that have been made both to users who participated and more widely (*dissemination and implementation*). The dissemination phase is a key aspect of a user involvement system, as it helps to spread good practice and is part of 'assisted wheel reinvention'.

We now find ourselves back where we started and need to consider a new aim for user involvement in the context of hospice services.

User involvement systems: co-ordination and sharing

Sharing user involvement experience between units and organisations, and co-ordinating service development, are key aspects of the system approach to user involvement.

Cancer services are complicated, and are composed of many different parts of the NHS and voluntary sector. They involve the provision of care by a range of health professionals. Typically, cancer services are organised around a cancer network which includes NHS hospitals, primary care trusts, voluntary organisations and local authorities, as well as strategic health authorities.

It is important that user involvement activities take place in all of the different contexts involved in cancer care. However, user involvement activities also need to be co-ordinated so that they feed into an overall user involvement system. Trusts will inevitably co-ordinate user involvement, but it may also be appropriate to look to the cancer network as a source of support and advice on user involvement activities.

Small-scale activities in a single setting can be important in user involvement. For example, a breast cancer clinic project – on exploring users' information needs about monitoring after treatment has finished – can contribute more broadly to service development. This type of project may have implications for the way in which other cancer services in a trust are organised. It may also influence the ways in which other members of the cancer network and other multidisciplinary teams think about how they provide information to their users.

Evaluating user involvement systems

National criteria

We have seen how it is increasingly important to be able to evaluate user involvement. The recent UK government publication *Involving Patients and the Public in Healthcare: a discussion document* (Department of Health, 2001) suggests several key principles underpinning public and patient empowerment.

These are as follows.

• Patients and the public are entitled to be involved wherever decisions are taken about care in the NHS.

- The involvement of patients and the public must be embedded in the structures of the NHS and permeate all aspects of healthcare.
- The public and patients should have access to relevant information.
- Healthcare professionals must be partners in the process of involving the public and patients.
- There must be honesty about the scope of the public's and patients' involvement, since some decisions cannot be made by the public.
- There must be transparency and openness in the procedures for involving the public and patients.
- The mechanisms for involvement should be evaluated for their effectiveness.
- The public and patients should have access to training and funding to allow them to participate fully.
- The public should be represented by a wide range of individuals and groups as well as by particular 'patient groups'.*

Other national sources of criteria for measuring the quality of user involvement include those adopted by the Commission for Health Improvement, the Audit Commission and the Scottish Executive Health Department. We have reproduced the Commission for Health Improvement Guidelines in the Appendix to Part 1.

The ASWCS criteria for evaluating user involvement

How we developed our criteria

Drawing on the Department of Health principles listed above, which were outlined in the Kennedy Report (2001), we have developed a set of criteria for the evaluation of user involvement within organisations.

To develop our criteria, we drew on a variety of sources:

- a range of literature
- data from interviews with 37 patients about user involvement in cancer services and 43 interviews with health professionals
- a formal consensus-building exercise involving input from 367 users, health service professionals or researchers
- case studies of particular organisations providing services to people with cancer across Avon, Somerset and Wiltshire.

---

*It is worth noting that this is misquoted from the Kennedy Report in the Department of Health Discussion paper and has been altered to reflect the original. For more information *see* Cancerlink 2001.

The ASWCS criteria

We shall now discuss in detail the criteria we developed in ASWCS to evaluate user involvement programmes.

We need to consider a range of different elements of user involvement when we are evaluating the user involvement process. In particular, we need to think about how each user involvement activity fits into a user involvement system. Thus a number of our criteria are about how mechanisms for involving users are part of a whole system of evaluating and developing service organisation and delivery. This means that individual one-off user involvement activities receive a lower rating than those that are part of a larger programme.

It is important to consider positive and negative aspects of what happens as the system develops, rather than simply to evaluate outcomes. The approach we have adopted seeks to do this by assessing whether a particular set of issues has not been developed, is currently being developed or is already in place. Our criteria can be helpful in pinpointing specific aspects of a user involvement system that need further development. The criteria themselves can also be helpful when designing a user involvement system.

The criteria encompass nine dimensions of user involvement:

A aims and scope of user involvement
B systematic approach to user involvement
C resources for user involvement
D information and communication
E training and support
F representation and inclusion
G power and control
H evidence of change
I feedback and follow-up.

These criteria are described fully in Part 2, Section 3G.

An assessment can be made for each criterion according to whether the organisation:

* has no plans to develop this element
* is currently developing this element
* already has this element in place.

We have set out a detailed example below showing how the criteria can be used.

Example: using the ASWCS criteria

This example from our research examines a hospital trust's Tumour-Specific User Group User Involvement Programme. Using criteria that the research team developed over the course of this study, we evaluated the User Involvement Programme and provided a report explaining what we found.

The evaluation process

The User Involvement Programme was based on collaboration with a local cancer voluntary organisation. The trust paid for seven of the organisation's volunteers to be trained as focus group facilitators. The notes of patients who had been diagnosed with a particular cancer type (tumour type) within the previous six months were extracted on a regular basis and sent to the relevant consultant to approve inclusion in the User Involvement Programme. Approved patients were sent a standard letter inviting them to attend a focus group at the hospital. They could bring a carer or friend if they wished. They were also asked to complete a brief questionnaire.

The focus group discussions were recorded and transcribed. Selections considered relevant by the User Group Facilitator were sent to the cancer manager, who further refined the report, and separated the aspects that were relevant to different Site Specialty Groups for circulation to the relevant consultants. The report was also circulated to members of the Cancer Services Review Group, which consisted of all the medical consultants treating cancer, the cancer leads from the local primary care groups, and the Deputy Lead Nurse.

The Cancer Services Review Group, chaired by the Trust's Cancer Lead Clinician, met to discuss and react to the report of the users' views gleaned from the questionnaires and focus groups.

The evaluation findings according to the ASWCS criteria

A Aims and scope of user involvement
Users were clearly defined as patients who had been diagnosed and treated for the specific cancer type during the previous 12 months, and their carers. The general aims of user involvement were made clear to individuals at the beginning of the focus group meeting. Not all of the procedures were clearly explained to or understood by everyone. For example, sometimes views that were expressed by users were treated as if they were complaints, even though the users themselves had not sought to complain. This was clearly problematic, and had a negative impact on the individual staff concerned as well as on overall staff morale.

Users' feedback was used in service development. Some changes were introduced in relation to users' retrospective accounts, but the goals and framework for making decisions were not always made clear. Thus there was a lack of systematic structures for taking decisions about action resulting from user involvement.

continued overleaf

Assessment: Overall, there was evidence that the aims of user involvement were stated and its scope considered. There was a need for further development in this area.

B Systematic approach to user involvement
The User Involvement Programme used focus groups of users as well as a questionnaire to elicit feedback. A series of focus groups was held for each tumour site, and a full cycle took about one year to complete.

Focus group discussions were transcribed and quotes were selected in order to draw attention to key issues. The rationale for this procedure was not clear to everyone. The full transcript of the focus group was not made readily available to all staff, and the results of the data analysis were not checked with the users. This introduced the risk that facilitators and managers may have attributed more or less importance to particular statements than that given by the users themselves.

Assessment: Overall, a systematic approach to user involvement was in place, but there were areas that needed further development. For example, users could have been consulted about the methods used to elicit feedback. The use of data and the validity of data analysis were also a concern.

C Resources for user involvement
The trust funded training for facilitators from the voluntary organisation. The User Involvement Facilitator was paid by the trust, although there was a query about whether payment met the full costs of time invested in the collection and analysis of data. Resources were not allocated to pay for clinical staff time to review the documents and participate in meetings of the Cancer Service Review Group.

Users were paid transport costs and, if necessary, childcare costs. Refreshments were provided at the meetings. There was an expectation that users would give their time freely.

Assessment: Overall, resources for user involvement were in place but could be developed.

D Information and communication
Users may have found out about the group through membership of local voluntary organisations, but there was little formal publicity. Users were told of the opportunity for user involvement in a letter inviting them to complete a questionnaire and attend a focus group. This meant that professionals could potentially prevent some users from taking part. For example, if a consultant or specialist nurse did not think that a user's involvement was appropriate, the user would not be sent the letter of invitation or become aware of user involvement opportunities.

continued opposite

Attempts were made to address users' communication needs, including their language and literacy needs as well as physical needs, although further steps could have been taken.

Participants were provided with feedback in the form of an annual letter summarising the impact of the User Involvement Programme on service development. However, there was no ongoing feedback for participants.

Informed consent* prior to participation was sought from those users who were involved. Formal written consent was not sought.

Assessment: Overall, information and communication issues were in the process of development. Improvements could be made in several areas, including providing access to involvement for users, addressing communication needs, informed consent and feedback to participants.

E Training and support
The trust paid for the training of facilitators from the voluntary organisation to facilitate the focus groups, but there was no training for other users or for staff. There was only limited support for users who attended a focus group, but there were advanced plans to build and develop a cancer information centre. There was no explicit support for involved users or staff, although informal support and counselling were available.

Assessment: Overall, training and support mechanisms were under development.

F Representation and inclusion
Recruitment was undertaken in a systematic fashion based on treated patients. However, this did not incorporate a mechanism for establishing the characteristics of those who were involved. The User Involvement Programme had input from voluntary organisations, but there did not appear to be any specific attempt to involve hard-to-reach individuals.

Assessment: Overall, representation and inclusion of diverse groups needed to be developed.

G Power and control
The user focus group's stated aim was to document users' experiences retro-spectively, and to highlight positive and negative aspects of their care. There was no clear mechanism for involving users directly in decisions about service development.

Staff attending the Cancer Services Review Group were informed about the User Involvement Programme but other staff did not appear to be informed about the user involvement groups and the reports of users' views.

continued overleaf

---

*Verbal consent based on being fully informed about what taking part means.

Assessment: Overall, power and control issues needed to be considered further and strategies developed. Key areas included consultation with users and staff about the methods and approach taken, data handling, and decisions taken on the basis of those data.

H Evidence of change
The user groups were held as part of an ongoing cycle. This was felt to provide an informal and indirect monitoring process. However, there was no systematic or regular review of the impact of user involvement on service delivery.

Assessment: Overall, informal mechanisms for providing evidence of change existed, but formal mechanisms may need to be developed.

I Feedback and follow-up
Users were provided with feedback in the form of an annual letter sent to those who participated in a focus group. This provided an account of the trust's key responses to issues that had been raised in groups, but it did not include a systematic response to all of the issues raised in the groups.

Assessment: Overall, feedback and follow-up mechanisms were in place, but could be further developed. For example, focus group participants could be invited to evaluate the outcome of the User Involvement Programme.

Frequently asked questions

Q: How do you measure quality in user involvement?

A: A number of aspects of user involvement relate to quality. We have suggested in this section how we approach quality. A key part of the measurement concerns how users feel about being involved, the extent of opportunities for user involvement, and the relationship between user involvement and outcomes.

Q: Who should evaluate a user involvement system?

A: It is important that the evaluation of the system should be done transparently – ideally this would involve both independent evaluators and users. More importantly, the evaluation should be fed back widely to the different parts and participants in the user involvement system, and any necessary changes should be made.

Q: Is the evaluation of user involvement objective?

A: Different users want different things from their involvement, just as an organisation may also have different aims for a user involvement system. The evaluation should examine ways in which the explicit aims of the involvement have been operationalised and the results put into practice. In addition, it must take account of the subjective experience of those who were involved, both users and health professionals.

Thus an evaluation should incorporate both subjective and objective measures. It should also aim to be comparable between sites and settings.

Q: How should the results of an evaluation be used?

A: The results of the evaluation should help to change the system to make it more responsive to users' views and better designed to ensure service and professional development. The results need to be fed back to the participants, users and health professionals to help them to change the way in which they approach user involvement, so that it will be more effective.

Q: Should an evaluation measure the process or outcome of user involvement?

A: User involvement is likely to identify specific issues that need to be addressed. An evaluation should identify what has been done to address these specific issues. This is part of an evaluation of the outcomes of a user involvement system.

However, involving users has an impact on the way in which a service is delivered, in that it changes the way in which service providers look at what they are doing. Thus user involvement is part of a process – not only of service development, but also of professional and personal development. Examining how a user involvement system has made an impact on personal and professional development is part of what an evaluation of the process of user involvement examines.

Q: What is the role of users in the evaluation?

A: Users should play a full part in the evaluation. Their particular insights will help to ensure that the system continues to respond to the needs and views of users.

References

- Department of Health (2001) *Involving Patients and the Public in Healthcare: a discussion document.* Department of Health, Leeds.

- Kennedy I (2001) *Learning from Bristol: the Report of the Public Inquiry into Children's Heart Surgery at the Bristol Royal Infirmary, 1984–1995.* The Stationery Office, London.

Further reading

- Beresford P and Croft S (1993) *Citizen Involvement: a practical guide for change.* Macmillan, London.

- Chambers R (1999) *Involving Patients and the Public.* Radcliffe Medical Press, Oxford.

- Commission for Health Improvement (2002) *'Nothing About Us Without Us': a patient and public strategy for the Commission for Health Improvement;* www.chi.nhs.uk/patients/index.shtml

- National Audit Office; www.nao.gov.uk

- National Institute for Clinical Excellence (NICE); www.nice.org.uk

- Office of Public Management and National Assembly for Wales (2001) *Signposts: a practical guide to public and patient involvement in Wales.* National Assembly for Wales, Cardiff.

SECTION 8

Implementation and dissemination

This section focuses on the *implementing and disseminating* stage of the cycle of user involvement.

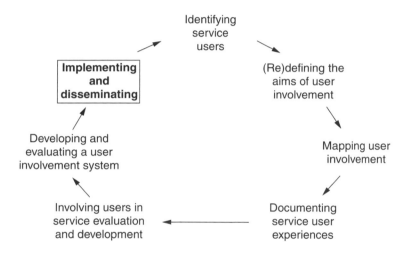

Cycle of user involvement.

In this section, we discuss:

- implementing changes that result from your user involvement work
- building a dissemination strategy
- dissemination methods – websites, newsletters, workshops and con-ferences
- examples of a briefing note, a press release and a project outline
- frequently asked questions.

Summary of key issues

- Implementation and dissemination are important, closely linked stages of the user involvement cycle.
- Implementation involves putting into practice the results of user involvement. Dissemination involves making sure that people know what those results are, whether or not changes take place.
- We discuss key issues that you need to consider when you implement change following user involvement activity, including feasibility and preparation. We also discuss a number of implementation strategies.
- Whether or not changes are introduced following user involvement, it is important to disseminate information about the process that has taken place and the decisions that have been made. Dissemination is important for several reasons – to complete the user involvement cycle, to develop a culture of user involvement, and to strengthen trust, accountability and partnership working.
- Key issues relating to dissemination include considering the message, the audience and the methods used.
- The section ends with a series of examples of dissemination methods, including websites, newsletters, stakeholder meetings, press releases and project summaries. All of these methods have been used successfully within the ASWCS project.

Introduction

Implementation is the process of putting the results of a user involvement activity into practice. It is also important to tell the right audience about the outcomes of user involvement – this is known as dissemination. This section focuses on these two closely related aspects of user involvement.

Implementation

Implementing changes initiated from a user involvement activity

The implementation of changes initiated from a user involvement activity is part of improving the services provided by your organisation. It is important to be clear why any proposed changes have or have not been implemented, and to feed back this information to service users and other stakeholders. This means that a user involvement activity should not just be a lip-service exercise – it should show respect for the people who have been involved and who feel that their contribution has made a difference.

Furthermore, at an organisational level you need to account for the use of time and resources invested in user involvement activities.

Some of the issues you need to consider when implementing a change are discussed below.

Feasibility of the change

How easy or difficult is it to implement this change?

At this stage you need to be able to answer questions such as what needs to be done and how you can make it happen. Furthermore, you should consider possible sources of help in order to implement change. You also need to take into account the budget and time implications of implementing change.

Pre-implementation preparation

Before developing an implementation strategy, it is helpful to analyse the possible outcomes of making the change, identifying all of the groups that could be affected. A formal (or informal) consultation with these groups can help you to assess how ready people are to accept change.

Key factors in the success of a proposed change are building a partnership and making a change seem less threatening. You should think about factors that might obstruct or promote the change – possible barriers to change (both external and internal), and how you could promote change with the right resources, skills and training.

Implementation strategies

There are different ways of implementing a change. For example, the *plan–do–study–act (PDSA) cycle* is a process model for quality improvement that has been used in health services. It consists of small-scale tests of planned actions, followed by assessment and improvement of the initial plan.

The success of an implementation strategy is dependent on the following factors:

- *leadership* – someone who will ensure that the project meets its targets
- *skills* – the right mix of people with appropriate skills to ensure that the change will take place
- *planning* – a flexible plan should also be in place, to ensure that a team can adapt to any unexpected issues
- *dissemination strategy* – you need to keep in touch with everyone who is affected by this work, so a good dissemination strategy is essential.

> **Examples of implementing change through a user involvement activity**
>
> **A feedback questionnaire**
> A feedback questionnaire on patient/carer experience was developed in conjunction with the clinical governance team at East Somerset NHS Trust.
>
> The questionnaire was given to all patients with a positive diagnosis of gynaecological and urological cancer, three months after diagnosis. Patients and carers were asked to comment on the service that they received.
>
> As a result of the first round of urology questionnaires, it was discovered that patients who were seen at peripheral clinics had no knowledge of or access to the Clinical Nurse Specialist for support or advice.
>
> This situation has now been remedied by ensuring that leaflets and contact cards are available at all peripheral urology clinics within the trust catchment area.
>
> **Interviews with service users**
> As part of the ASWCS user involvement project, we conducted interviews with ten prostate cancer service users at United Bristol Health Care Trust.
>
> Three service users expressed a need for a support group for prostate cancer patients in the Bristol area.
>
> As a result, with assistance from the multidisciplinary team, a support group has been running in the Bristol area since April 2002.

Building a dissemination strategy

Why disseminate?

The word 'dissemination' comes from the Latin *disseminare*, which means to sow. In other words, dissemination is about distributing publicity on the outcomes of your work so that good practice can grow elsewhere. People usually put a lot of time and effort into their user involvement methodology, without necessarily doing the same for dissemination of the results.

Dissemination is more than just producing a good final report. It implies that what you have done is reaching everyone who should be aware of your activity or who will benefit from what you have achieved.

There are a number of reasons why dissemination is so important.

- *Completing a user involvement cycle.* Dissemination feeds the outcomes of an involvement activity into the user involvement cycle. It could also result in the identification of further possible user involvement work.
- *Developing a user involvement culture.* You can communicate good practice by increasing awareness of the outcomes of your user involvement

activities. By targeting the right audience, you can influence others to make use of your methodology and avoid any pitfalls that you may have encountered.

- *Accountability*. Accountability can be seen as an agreement or exchange between two parties in which essentially one says 'You give me the means and I will do what we agreed upon,' and the other says 'Fine, so long as you demonstrate that you are doing it well.' Good dissemination can ensure the accountability of what you are trying to achieve.
- *Building partnerships with service users*. User involvement can go one step further by engaging service users in the organisation of workshops or conferences. This can forge partnerships with services, which can be very useful for developing future user involvement initiatives. Service users can become involved in making presentations or facilitating work- shops at conferences. For example, at the ASWCS conference for launching the consensus statement, the service user representative was one of the speakers in the plenary session. There are also examples of users success- fully running a whole event, such as the annual conference of cancer self- help groups.
- *Engaging with multiple stakeholders*. Reasons why you may want to engage with people outside your unit or organisation include the following.
  - You may want to make sure that what you have done fits into the bigger picture.
  - Other people may want to repeat what you have done in a different context.
  - You may have produced a questionnaire for cancer patients, but it could be useful for people with other conditions.
  - It can have a 'buddying' effect, so that you can share experiences with other people who work in this field.

Dissemination is more than just a public relations exercise. It ensures that the results of your user involvement activities are made public and add to what is known in your field. In order to be more effective, you need to develop a dissemination strategy.

Key issues for a dissemination strategy

You need to consider a number of issues in order to develop an effective and consistent dissemination strategy.

The importance of the message

You may have spent quite a few months working on a project. You might be clear in your mind how the outcomes of your project fit with what is known in the field and how it could improve services. However, this is not necessarily clear to other people.

You should decide on a key message that you want people to take away. It may be useful to consider how what you have found out fits with what is already known. For example, in the *British Medical Journal* an article may have a text box next to the introduction describing briefly what is already known in the relevant field.

Make your message user friendly

We live in an era of information overload – just consider how many emails, letters or phone calls you receive during your working day. Your message needs to be as clear and simple as possible. A newsletter can be useful, or you could consider producing a toolkit or guidelines for people working in this field, based on the results of your study.

The importance of the audience

Once you have decided what you want to talk about, it is crucial to consider what audience it is for. Is it for healthcare professionals? Is it for the service users? The audience you want to target will influence the choice of dissemination methods.

If you want to influence health professionals, you may want to use a professional journal such as the *British Medical Journal*, the *Nursing Times* or the *Health Services Journal*. You could disseminate your results by presenting them at a scientific conference, or you could consider the local press or a national newspaper such as the *Guardian* if you want to influence a larger audience. Alternatively, you may want to get in touch with different stakeholders, in which case a workshop or a conference might be more effective.

Engaging the users

Service users should be an integral part of any dissemination strategy. Users can be engaged from the beginning of a user involvement project, as their input can be paramount in developing a strategy that is relevant to the local community. A newsletter, an Internet web page and the creative use of media are essential in this case.

Dissemination methods

We shall now focus on different dissemination methods. We shall discuss in detail the development of a website and the creation of a newsletter;

these can be useful ways of reaching a wide audience, especially service users. We also include examples of the use of other media.

A website

The Internet is a network that connects computers around the world. It is quite an effective way of disseminating your user involvement activity. More and more people nowadays have a presence on the Web, and many people use the Internet to find information.

Why have a website?

The Internet is often a more effective way of disseminating your outcomes than a traditional paper report, which might just sit on a library shelf. A website can help you to reach a wider audience, and its interactive nature means that you can use it to obtain feedback on your involvement activity.

When might a website not be useful?

A website is not useful if you are working on something that you do not want in the public domain. Also, although increasing numbers of people have access to the Internet, you may still be unable to reach some groups, such as disadvantaged people.

Summary of the advantages and disadvantages of a website

Advantages
- Reaches a wider audience – both healthcare professionals and service users
- Can be used at all stages of the user involvement cycle
- Adaptable – can be up to date, focusing on the latest developments in your activity

Disadvantages
- Time and resources implications – you may need training in or assistance with web-page editing
- Can be problematic if you are working on something confidential
- People tend to forget copyright when it comes to Internet material, and use it without acknowledging its source
- It may exclude people who do not have access to the Internet

---

When to use a website

A web page can be useful at all stages of the user involvement cycle. It is an effective way of communicating, especially if several organisations are involved. You can obtain feedback on your research, or you can even use your website as a research tool. For example, you could consider including an electronic version of a questionnaire, or conducting a Delphi exercise by email.

Resources you need: checklist for websites

Equipment/resource	*Tasks and things to consider*
Software package	FrontPage Editor is the most commonly used software. You may need training or someone to assist you with this process
Finance	You might need to pay for software/training or assistance
Host for your web page	Does your organisation have an Internet presence or do you need a commercial provider?

How to develop a website

This is a summary of how to go about setting up a website (for a more detailed description of what is involved, *see* Part 2, Section 2F).

How to develop a website: summary of procedure

1 Define your aims	Be clear about what you want to achieve by setting up a website
2 Design the site	Good design is crucial, and you may want expert help with this
3 Go online	The technicalities of 'uploading' your website to the Internet
4 Make it happen	There a number of ways to attract people to your website
5 Update your site	Most websites need to be regularly updated in order to get people to revisit them

Example: user involvement project website

The following is an example of the ASWCS user involvement project home page (www.aswcs.nhs.uk/aswcs/DoH/doh.htm). It gives an overview of the project, and by following the links you can find further information. There are clear links both to the project newsletter and to another page that provides information on how people can become involved.

DoH User Involvement Research	**Avon, Somerset and Wiltshire NHS** Cancer Services
Up Project Outline How Can I Get Involved? Newsletter November 2001 Main Menu Home Contact Us Primary Care Hospital Services Hospices Support Organisations Standards of Care Web Links Feedback Site Map Search	Developing and Evaluating Best Practice for User Involvement in Cancer Services Project Summary This project is reviewing current practice for involving users in the development of cancer services. User involvement can mean many different things, from involving patients in decisions about their care to involving patients and carers in organisational decisions and development. The project focus is on the general development of cancer services. For further information please follow the links below Project Outline How Can I Get Involved

Newsletters

A newsletter is a good way of keeping in touch with people who have participated or showed an interest in your user involvement activity. Although this section refers to developing your own newsletter, you could also publicise your activity by contributing to existing newsletters.

Why develop a newsletter?

A newsletter is a good way of keeping in touch with people who have been involved in your project. You can update them on progress, and it is a way of giving them feedback. You can also use it to share your findings with a wider audience.

When might newsletters not be useful?

It is important to be clear about the audience for your newsletter, as its format must accommodate their needs. If a newsletter would not meet their needs, it is obviously not a useful thing to produce.

Summary of the advantages and disadvantages of newsletters

Advantages
- Effective way of disseminating your results to a wider community
- Accountability – giving feedback to people who have been involved

Disadvantages
- A lot of preparation is needed – it can be quite time consuming and resource intensive
- Can exclude people whose first language is not English

When should you produce a newsletter?

A newsletter could be useful at any point of the user involvement cycle. You could produce one at the start of a user involvement activity, to increase awareness about your project and to recruit volunteers, or you could use it later on to give feedback to people who have been involved.

Resources you need: checklist for newsletters

Equipment/resource	*Tasks and things to consider*
Finance	Desktop publishing software, publishing the newsletter
Administration	Sending out the newsletter

How to develop a newsletter

The table below provides a summary of how you might go about developing a newsletter (for a more detailed description, *see* Part 2, Section 2G).

How to develop a newsletter: summary of procedure

1	Define your aims	Be clear about what you want your newsletter to achieve
2	Design the newsletter	The format and language of the newsletter will depend largely on your intended audience
3	Get it printed	Will this be done in-house or commercially, and what will it cost?
4	Distribute it	Who is your newsletter for and how will they obtain it?
5	Evaluate it	Make sure that your readers can give you comments and suggestions

Example: table of contents of a newsletter

The following extract is taken from the ASWCS user involvement project newsletter. The table of contents shows the principles behind a good newsletter.

- The intended audience for the newsletter is evident (service users and health professionals).
- The different sections of the newsletter are clearly signposted.
- Readers have an opportunity to comment via a contact person.

Table of contents of ASWCS newsletter

Welcome to our second newsletter for health service users and healthcare professionals.

In this issue

The consensus statement conference	page 1
Action points from the conference workshop	page 2
User involvement: is it satisfying?	page 3
Our new web pages	page 4
How to get involved	page 4

We welcome your feedback: please send any comments or suggestions about this newsletter to AN Other at xxxxxxxxx

Meetings with stakeholders (workshops or conferences)

Workshops can provide a forum where people can define and solve problems. The organisation of workshops has already been discussed in Part 1, Section 6, but we have set out below an example of a workshop that was organised to launch the consensus statement that ASWCS developed.

The programme tried to obtain a balance between plenary sessions and group activities. The morning focused on the launch of the *Toolkit*, and there were three sessions of workshops in which people could give feedback. In the first workshop, people were asked to divide up according to their professional groups to discuss the implications of the consensus statement for their professional practice. In the later workshops, delegates had an opportunity to discuss specific issues raised by the consensus statement and to interact with people from different backgrounds. They could attend two different afternoon workshops, as they were both run twice.

Example: ASWCS workshop programme to launch consensus statement

09.30	Coffee
10.00	Welcome and Introduction
10.10	Presentation on the Health in Partnership (HiP) initiative
10.30	Promoting user involvement: the voluntary sector perspective. User involvement in cancer services: a personal experience
11.00	Questions and Discussion
11.10	Coffee Break
11.30	Developing the consensus statement on best practice in user involvement in cancer services
11.55	Implementing the consensus statement: implications for service development
12.15	Workshop Session 1: Opportunities and constraints for implementing user involvement in cancer services

	Group 1a	Clinicians
	Group 1b	Managers
	Group 1c	Nurses and Professions Allied to Medicine (PAMs)
	Group 1d	Service Users/User Groups
	Group 1e	Cancer Education Professionals

13.00	Lunch Break
14.15	Workshop Session 2/3: Developing best practice in user involvement: key themes

	Group 2a	Aims, scope and benefits of user involvement
	Group 2b	The role of information and communication in user involvement

continued opposite

	Group 2c	Developing effective methods of user involvement
	Group 2d	Training and support for user involvement
	Group 2e	Resources for user involvement
15.15	Final Session: Main issues raised during workshop sessions
16.30	Close

Examples of the use of different media

Finally, we provide some examples of different ways to disseminate your results. These are not by any means exhaustive, and are no substitute for formal training in media and writing skills.

As part of a dissemination strategy you have to remember the importance of your message and the audience that you want to reach – note the difference in language and style depending on the audience. Consultation with service users is always helpful.

- The first example is a briefing note intended for a policy document. It is an executive summary of the first-year results of the ASWCS user involvement project, aimed at policy makers.
- The second example is a press release for the consensus statement, which we sent to the local press.
- The third example is the first page of a project outline, aimed at a more academic audience.

Example 1: a briefing note

Avon, Somerset and Wiltshire Cancer Services (ASWCS) have been awarded a grant under the Department of Health's *Health in Partnership* initiative to develop and evaluate best practice for user involvement in cancer services. This research is a collaborative project with the University of the West of England (UWE), the University of Warwick, Bristol Cancer Help Centre and Cancerlink.

Initial research activities have included a questionnaire, which was sent to healthcare commissioners and providers across ASWCS, as well as to voluntary sector groups with a focus on or interest in cancer. The questionnaire focused on structural issues with regard to user involvement in the different organisations.

A series of structured meetings using the nominal group technique (NGT) have also taken place. The aim of these meetings was to explore agreed themes in order to develop a consensus statement for user involvement. The groups involved healthcare professionals and health service managers, as well as patients and their carers.

continued overleaf

The initial findings suggest that there is widespread support for user involvement across the statutory and voluntary sectors. However, there is not clear agreement as to what user involvement actually is.

There is also wide variation in user involvement experience and approaches across organisations. In the statutory sector, user involvement is more advanced in local councils or community health councils (CHCs) compared with cancer services providers.

The main barriers to a more widespread range of user involvement in the voluntary sector seem to be the organisational diversity of this sector and the difficulty in motivating hard-to-reach social groups.

Analysis of the nominal groups generated ten themes relating to user involvement in cancer services:

- the aims of user involvement
- the scope of user involvement
- the infrastructure and resources for user involvement
- the culture of user involvement
- information/communication issues
- representation and inclusion considerations
- methods of user involvement
- recognising users' experiences and addressing users' needs
- training and support for user involvement
- feedback and implementation.

These themes will be key to the process of consensus development. The data collected also contain insights about the nature of professional interaction and how professional cultures might affect the implementation of user involvement strategies.

These findings will be widely disseminated via the ASWCS network, and the consensus statement will be launched in autumn 2001. Furthermore, issues for action arising from this research exercise will be identified. The next stage of the research focuses on developing a tool to measure satisfaction with user involvement. The project runs until September 2002.

Example 2: a press release

Cancer patients' power endorsed
Avon, Somerset and Wiltshire Cancer Services has set out a statement on how they will ensure that patients have a key voice in evaluating and developing cancer services. It is part of a research project funded by the Department of Health in collaboration with the University of the West of England, Warwick University, Bristol Cancer Help Centre and Cancerlink.

continued opposite

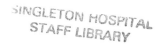
'Involving patients or cancer service users is really key to our work in improving cancer services. We have now set out in a consensus statement some basic principles of how we will do it', said James Rimmer, Director of Avon, Somerset and Wiltshire Cancer Services, which is a collaborative network of local organisations working to improve cancer care.

The consensus statement was put together following wide consultation with doctors, managers, nurses, the voluntary sector, researchers and cancer service users. Nine statements about user involvement have received universal support from all of the participants.

The statements are as follows.

- The aim of user involvement is to improve cancer services.
- Users should be able to be involved in decisions about their care.
- To get users involved, there must be a willingness of professionals to accept users' participation.
- There should be a good organisational system to support user involvement.
- It should be clear to everyone why they are taking part in user involvement.
- It is important to give feedback to users who have been consulted.
- All users' communication needs should be addressed, including those arising from language, physical and psychological difficulties.
- Information about opportunities for user involvement should be provided as part of general information on cancer services.
- There should be a variety of methods available that meet users' practical and emotional needs.

'Involving patients and service users is vital in helping us improve cancer services. We believe this statement is pioneering in that it sets out the reality of how we will involve users at every stage', said James Rimmer.

Example 3: a project outline: first page

Health in Partnership Project 12: Developing and evaluating best practice for user involvement in cancer services

Introduction
This project, funded by the Department of Health, is reviewing current practice for involving users in the development of cancer services. The project is a collaboration between Avon, Somerset and Wiltshire Cancer Services (ASWCS, an accredited cancer network), the University of the West of England and the University of Warwick. The project team also includes members drawn from the Bristol Cancer Help Centre and Cancerlink, as well as designated user representatives.

continued overleaf

User involvement can mean many different things, from involving patients in decisions about their care to involving patients and carers in organisational decisions and development. We are interested in all of these aspects, but our main emphasis is on the general development of cancer services.

The research project has four key objectives:

- to map existing activity and examples of user involvement across ASWCS
- to develop a statement, agreed by a wide range of participants, identifying key priorities for the development of user involvement in cancer services. This is known as a consensus statement
- to develop a questionnaire to assess patients' perspectives on ways in which they would like to be involved in service development, and to find out how satisfied patients and carers are with their current experiences of involvement. This questionnaire will be used with different groups in order to find out about a range of experiences. We shall be particularly interested in the experiences of patients cared for by professionals who have received education and training in user involvement
- to develop a toolkit incorporating models of best practice and methods of enhancing user involvement in the development of cancer services.

Frequently asked questions

Q: What is the added value of getting users involved in the dissemination strategy?

A: Service users should be part of your dissemination process so that you can ensure that the process is relevant to them. Different dissemination events, such as workshops or conferences, mean that health professionals and service users can interact outside the boundaries of a clinical consultation. The experience is enlightening for both groups.

Q: What type of feedback do I need to give to service users who have been involved?

A: It is important to give feedback to users – not just out of courtesy – thanking them for sparing some of their time to get involved. The accountability of the whole user involvement exercise depends on giving feedback.

Feedback can be in the form of a letter, a newsletter or a workshop – you will have to decide on the best way to inform the people whom you have consulted. In any case, your message should clearly state the outcome of the user involvement initiative. If you have been unable to take on board the recommendations of the service users with whom you worked, you should explain the reasons for this clearly.

Q: How can I know that my dissemination strategy has been successful?

A: The only way to find out whether your dissemination strategy has been successful is to check with the people who participated. A feedback form to allow these individuals to comment on the event can be very useful.

Q: How can I make sure that the information I present is easily accessible?

A: Your information should be appropriate for the audience that you want to reach. Your newsletter or feedback letter should be written in plain English. 'Plain English' is defined as something that the intended audience can read, understand and act upon the first time they read it. It takes into account design and layout as well as language.

Q: How can I disseminate the user involvement results to hard-to-reach groups?

A: Your dissemination process should be inclusive. You should try to reach out to these communities, rather than expect them to contact you. Dedicating resources to outreach work can be an effective way of contacting service users from more marginalised groups, such as older people or individuals from minority ethnic groups. Personal contact is much more effective than letters and leaflets. The assistance of community leaders can be crucial here. You should also be aware of any cultural and religious needs that may affect the involvement of hard-to-reach groups.

Further reading

- Langley C, Nolan K, Nolan T, Norman C and Provost L (1996) *The Improvement Guide: a practical approach to improving organisational performance.* Jossey-Bass Publishers, San Francisco, CA.

- NHS Centre for Reviews and Dissemination (1999) *Effective Health Care: bulletin on the effectiveness of health service interventions for decision makers.* Volume 5. NHS Centre for Reviews and Dissemination, University of York, York.

Professional education and training for user involvement

In this section, we discuss:

- reasons why health professionals sometimes find it difficult to work together
- the challenges of interprofessional education and criteria for success
- two case studies of interprofessional education
- key elements for successful professional education for user involvement.

Summary of key issues

- If user involvement is to become part of the everyday culture of health services, it is likely that specialist education and training will be needed for both health professionals and service users.
- Service users may contribute to multidisciplinary education and training. They may also have additional needs for education and training in user involvement, as well as support, while going through the involvement process. You should consider users' needs for training and support on an ongoing basis at each stage of the cycle of user involvement.
- User involvement is unlikely to develop effectively without professional education and training. Research has shown that a lack of collaboration between professionals can have a negative effect on patients, and can limit the scope of user involvement.
- Interprofessional education is a useful way to improve collaboration between professionals as well as to enhance user involvement. Although most interprofessional education projects are focused on professionals, service users can contribute useful expertise.
- We discuss the challenges of interprofessional education in user involvement, focusing on two case studies in the ASWCS network. Drawing on this experience, we suggest that there are a number of prerequisites for effective professional education, including a shared understanding of the meaning of user involvement, as well as support and encouragement for both professionals and users.

continued overleaf

> • Although professionals taking part should not be allowed to opt out of working with service users directly, it is important to recognise the fears and anxieties that professionals may experience when they approach service users to discuss service evaluation and development issues.

Introduction

Although health professionals are all working towards the same goal of delivering high-quality services, they sometimes find it difficult to work together. Yet lack of collaboration between professionals can create difficulties for service users and can severely limit the scope of user involvement.

The reasons why professionals do not always work together effectively include lack of knowledge and understanding about each others' roles, particularly if their training has taken place in isolation from other groups and from service users. Other issues, such as elitism and rivalry between professionals, can also get in the way of effective collaboration.

Interprofessional education

Interprofessional education aims to involve people from different professional groups in a process of shared learning, and to encourage teamwork.

Working together

For user involvement to succeed, you are likely to need collaboration between a range of professionals as well as between professionals and users.

Providing interprofessional education and training is, in practice, complex and challenging, especially if the focus is to increase user involvement in service development. The following difficulties can arise.

- It might be difficult to recruit some professional groups, particularly doctors, to interprofessional training.
- User involvement is likely to be one of a number of aims, as professionals have a range of educational needs.
- Professionals may be reluctant to engage with users, partly because of fears about what users might say, but also because they do not want to put their patients under any kind of pressure to give feedback.

Educating for successful user involvement

If education and training programmes are to successfully encourage user involvement, the following criteria need to be met.

- You need a shared understanding of the meaning of user involvement, including direct and indirect user involvement.
- Participants need to gain an understanding of a range of methods of user involvement.
- Professionals taking part need support and encouragement in their efforts to engage with service users.
- Service users taking part need support and adequate information about services and professional roles.
- Participants should not be able to opt out of working with service users directly.
- Ethical concerns should be addressed and all procedures should be clearly explained.

The issue of professional education for user involvement was a major element of the ASWCS project. We found that when we met these criteria, both users and professionals gained direct benefits from education and training. Education and training can improve communication between users and professionals as well as increasing users' information about services. Without this type of support, professionals are unlikely to involve service users willingly or effectively.

Case studies: education for user involvement

Case study 1: The Interprofessional Cancer Education Project (IPCE)
This project ran concurrently with the Department of Health User Involvement Project (and was intended to link in with it to some extent), and was supported by an initiative of the (then) South and West Regional Health Authority.

It involved working with healthcare teams and educating them to use a quality-improvement tool to implement change, during which process they had to involve users.

This was a structured educational programme that led to participants achieving academic credits.

One of the key findings was the difficulty that professionals experienced in actually engaging with users as colleagues in developing services. For example, one participant said:

> I have been working in the NHS for 20 years and I have never had discussions of this type with patients.
>
> (IPCE project, nurse year 1)

continued overleaf

It was apparent that professionals felt a lack of confidence in approaching patients, and sometimes felt unsupported by senior colleagues. Sometimes they seemed to be at odds with the policies of the NHS trust in which they worked, or they encountered a requirement to seek ethical approval when in fact their initiative could be run as an audit project.

In order to address these issues, we introduced a formal educational component to support the work-based learning, to help the teams to engage with users. This was subsequently formally incorporated into the programme, which was eventually mainstreamed into the Faculty MA module. (Details of this module, and associated modules at levels 2 and 3, can be obtained from the Faculty of Health and Social Care at the University of the West of England.)

Not everyone needs or wants academic credits, and for some the very idea can be a complete turn-off! Nevertheless, we were aware that the problem of engaging with users remained for all those professionals in the field who were required to do so. We found that the same issues were arising for the multidisciplinary teams within the network. Our realisation of this led to the further project, 'Promoting Best Practice in User Involvement' (PBPUI), which is described in more detail below.

Case study 2: Promoting Best Practice in User Involvement (PBPUI)
(A more detailed description of this programme can be found in Part 2, Section 2I.)

We recruited 'professional mentors' to work with teams. The mentors were individuals experienced in user involvement, who we had canvassed to elicit their active participation.

We provided a small amount of money (about £500) for each of the teams to help them carry out their plans. This was used for things such as printing and distributing a questionnaire, providing refreshments and travel expenses for a meeting involving patients, or developing a patient information leaflet.

The programme had five stages:

- *stage 1* – an introductory workshop
- *stage 2* – teams identified one simple issue they would like to work on
- *stage 3* – a second workshop lasting a whole day, so that the teams could give feedback about their progress, tell us about their issues, and plan what they wanted to do over the next six months
- *stage 4* – teams carried out their work on the identified issue. An essential component of this stage was that the teams actively involved users and worked with them in some way
- *stage 5* – a final workshop in which groups were asked to present what they had been doing in the form of a simple presentation or poster.

continued opposite

Evaluation

In both of the projects described in these case studies, the educational initiatives helped the multidisciplinary teams to involve their users in addressing some aspect of service development. The most striking aspects of the programme evaluations were that:

- the teams so profoundly needed this type of structured facilitation to give them sufficient confidence to engage with users
- they found the experience so deeply satisfying.

One of the IPCE team members commented:

> The thing that I learnt very much was that learning by practice and relating theory, although I learnt this at university, seeing it in action was very beneficial because it does work, because these lessons I'll carry forever now. I've learnt something that won't be taken away.
>
> (IPCE project, team member)

The educational process

Co-operation between organisations

An important element of the educational process was that it was a co-operative venture between the cancer network management and the local higher education provider, namely the University of the West of England (UWE).

Different organisations have different skills and qualities, and in this instance a key component of success was that we drew together expertise in user involvement from the university (a lecturer who had recognised skills) and a senior manager in the network. The lecturer had direct contact with the teams and also had responsibility for accreditation. Thus she was aware that teams were going to need to demonstrate how they had worked with users, and she could encourage them to take advantage of this opportunity for support. Her wide links across the network also allowed her to identify individuals who might be able to provide mentorship support, and invite them to participate.

A final member of the team, whose main work was in the cancer voluntary sector, provided additional expertise and encouragement, and perhaps had more flexibility within her role to provide additional liaison between the network and the university. Neither the university nor the network could have achieved the educational initiative without this kind of collaboration.

Learning in teams

Both projects (IPCE and PBPUI) took place over approximately an academic year. In both projects it was teams, rather than individuals, who we invited to participate. A relevant point for anyone else trying to institute the same process is that team selection should to some extent reflect the organisational structure on the ground. In the case of our local network, the initiative was aimed at the multidisciplinary teams for different cancer specialities.

We also recognised that any process of change requires senior members of the team to be 'on board', even if other people actually carry out the work.

Key elements for success

It is clear to us that educating professionals to involve users is an essential component of the process of actually implementing user involvement policy.

In our work, key elements for success were as follows:

- the involvement of teams rather than individuals
- the support of management within participating organisations
- some additional resources as a 'carrot', available as 'ring-fenced' but conditional on active engagement with users
- collaboration between the academic or skilled practitioner in user involvement, and the cancer network management
- a clear structured process, simply described with the necessary forms and tools (such as an audit tool) provided for the teams
- support in the field from skilled mentors
- the policy context within which the requirement to engage with users is 'non-negotiable'
- 'rewards and strokes' in the sense of recognition and achievement for participating teams.

A final key aspect is that if you want to effect real change in the area of user involvement, you need to appreciate that it is not completely 'resource neutral', although it does not need to involve vast expense. Our provision of a small amount of ring-fenced funding helped to unify and assist the process. In the case of the PBPUI project, it was £10 000 – averaging rather less than £1000 per multidisciplinary team, including facilitation fees to the university.

In summary, the type of education required is a process of what might be termed 'informed hand-holding'. This is a blend of theoretical and practical support. It is accompanied by the carrot of resources, within a context of formal requirement to engage with the issues, (e.g. the need to comply with accreditation processes). The two case studies we described above illustrate one model, which was not without problems of implementation, but which overall was successful. It is one essential component of the toolkit for user involvement.

Further reading

- Barr H (2002) *Interprofessional Education Today, Yesterday and Tomorrow. Centre for Health Sciences and Practice. Occasional Paper No. 1.* Centre for the Advancement of Interprofessional Education, London.

- Barr H and Waterton S (1996) *Interprofessional Education in Health and Social Care in the United Kingdom. Report of a CAIPE Survey.* Centre for the Advancement of Interprofessional Education, London.

- Daykin N, Rimmer J *et al.* (2002) Enhancing user involvement through interprofessional education: the case of cancer services. *Learning in Health and Social Care.* **13**: 122–31.

- Leathard A (1994) *Going Interprofessional. Working together for health and welfare.* Routledge, London.

- Turton PH and Holman H (2002) *Improving the Quality of Cancer Care: a team-based cancer education programme. Final evaluation.* Avon, Somerset and Wiltshire Cancer Services/University of the West of England, Bristol.

- Zwarenstein M, Atkins J, Barr H, Hammick M, Koppel I and Reeves S (1999) A systematic review of interprofessional education. *J Interprof Care.* **13**: 417–29.

Ethical issues

In this section, we discuss:

- ethical practice in user involvement, especially treating people with respect and providing support
- informed consent
- handling data
- research ethics committees – whether you need to approach them, and if so, how.

Summary of key issues

- It is essential to ensure that everyone who participates in user involvement activities acts ethically and follows principles of good practice.
- The central ethical concern in user involvement is about ensuring that the people involved are treated with respect and have access to appropriate support if they feel upset by the process.
- This section provides a general discussion of ethical principles in user involvement, including issues of informed consent and data handling. We provide an example of good practice in user involvement research, and a specimen information sheet for involved users.
- This section ends with a discussion of the role of research ethics committees in user involvement. Most user involvement is not classed as research but as service development. However, there may be cases where you require the approval of an ethics committee.
- Our project experience has shown that some professionals are daunted by applying for approval from an ethics committee. Yet this should not be used as a reason for avoiding involving users – failure to involve users in service development can also be seen as breaching an important ethical principle.

Introduction

The way in which users are involved has a direct effect on how they feel about the NHS and the particular organisation that contacted them. It is essential to ensure that all those who participate in user involvement activities act ethically and follow principles of good practice.

What is ethical practice?

The central concern of ethics in user involvement is about ensuring that the people involved are treated with respect. User involvement should not harm participants, and there should be appropriate support mechanisms in place for users who feel upset by the process.

An example of good practice when involving service users

Members of the project team undertook research to identify what cancer patients and carers felt their needs were for support and self-management (Barley *et al.*, 1999).

Data were collected using focus groups. All of the focus groups had both a facilitator and a co-facilitator. One of the key tasks of the co-facilitator was to provide support for participants who became upset. When this occurred, the co-facilitator was able to take them to a separate area and sit down and talk with them. This provided a way of helping people to manage their emotional reactions to the research without excluding them. In the few cases where this happened, after talking with the co-facilitator for a few minutes the participant rejoined the focus group and continued to take part in the discussion.

When preparing for the focus group, we put together an information pack for participants. This pack included local, regional and national addresses, telephone numbers and websites of key sources of information and support for people affected by cancer (e.g. CancerBACUP and the local Cancer Information Centre). This meant that all of the participants had ways of obtaining help if they became upset later on.

Informed consent

A key issue relates to 'informed consent'. This means that:

- users are volunteers and are asked to participate
- before any user involvement activities occur all of the users know how they will be involved, the types of methods that will be used and how the data that relate to them will be handled
- users have the right to withdraw (to cease being involved) at any time, and no one should be pressurised to become involved.

You should give potentially involved users a written information sheet that provides sufficient information to allow them to decide whether they want to take part. You should also give users a consent form to sign, indicating that they understand the nature of the user involvement exercise and agree to participate.

It is particularly important to consider that many users are also patients and are dependent on the NHS for their continued healthcare. This dependency can make them reluctant to refuse to participate, or to be critical of those who have cared for them in the past or might do so in the future.

Obtaining real informed consent is difficult for users who cannot speak for themselves (e.g. the very young). With such categories of users, including mentally ill people, children and users with learning difficulties, it is important to take particular care to be sure that they understand what they are agreeing to. Similarly, for users who do not speak English or who have communication difficulties, you must take care to provide information about user involvement activities in a form that they can understand. It is important that written information about user involvement is as non-technical and easy to understand as possible.

Suggested contents of a user involvement information sheet

1   *Title of study*
    The title should be clear and self-explanatory to a lay person.*
2   *Invitation to take part*
    This should explain that the user is being asked to take part in a user involvement exercise. The following is a suitable example:

> You are being invited to take part in a user involvement exercise. Before you decide it is important for you to understand why we are doing this and what it will involve. Please take time to read the following information carefully and discuss it with others if you wish. Ask us if anything is not clear or if you would like more information. Take time to decide whether or not you wish to take part.
>
> Thank you for reading this.

3   *What is the purpose of the user involvement exercise?*
    The background and aim of the user involvement exercise should be stated here. Both the extent to which the outcomes will change services and the limitations should be made explicit.
4   *Why have I been chosen?*
    You should explain how the user was chosen and how many other users will take part in the user involvement exercise.
5   *Do I have to take part?*
    You should explain that participation in the user involvement exercise is entirely voluntary. You could use the following paragraph:

> It is up to you to decide whether or not to take part. If you do decide to take part, you will be given this information sheet to keep and be asked to sign a consent form. If you decide to take part

continued overleaf

---

*A lay person is someone who does not have specialist knowledge or experience.

you are still free to withdraw at any time and without giving a reason. A decision to withdraw at any time, or a decision not to take part, will not affect the standard of care you receive.

6 *What will happen to me if I take part?*
You should state how long the user involvement exercise will last and how long the user will be involved. You should explain whether the user will need to attend meetings, where and when these will take place and whether travel expenses are available. What exactly will happen in the user involvement exercise (interviews, focus groups, etc.)? What are the users' responsibilities? Explain clearly what you expect of them.

7 *What will happen to the findings?*
You should state how you are going to feed back the findings of the user involvement exercise to participants, including a date when this will happen.

8 *Will my participation in this study be kept confidential?*
You should explain that all information collected about the user will be kept strictly confidential. A suggested form of words is as follows:

> All information which is collected about you during the course of the user involvement exercise will be kept strictly confidential. Any information about you that leaves the hospital/surgery will have your name and address removed so that you cannot be recognised from it.

You should always bear in mind that you, as the researcher, are responsible for ensuring that when collecting or using data you are not contravening the legal or regulatory requirements in any part of the UK.

9 *What will happen to the results of the user involvement exercise?*
You should be able to tell the patients what will happen to the results of the user involvement exercise. When are the results likely to be made public? Where can they obtain a copy of the results? You might add that they will not be identified in any report/publication.

10 *Who is organising and funding the user involvement exercise?*
The answer to this question should include the organisation that is sponsoring, funding or participating in the user involvement exercise (e.g. Medical Research Council, NHS trust, voluntary organisation or charity, academic institution).

11 *Contact for further information and final details*
You should give the user a contact point for further information. This can be your name or that of another person who is involved in the user involvement exercise.

12 *Remember to thank the user for taking part in the exercise*
The user information sheet should be dated and given a version number. This sheet should state that the user will be given a copy of the information sheet and a signed consent form to keep.

Respecting involved users

Respect in user involvement must go further. It is also about:

- providing ongoing feedback to users about the consequences and out-comes of their involvement
- being clear and open about the limitations of the methods used
- being clear about the potential for user involvement to make a difference.

Handling data

User involvement is personal – people participate in user involvement activities and give part of themselves to that process. Often users will utilise their own experience as a basis for their involvement, so the data that emerge from user involvement activities are personal data. It is important that the confidentiality of users is maintained.

It is good practice not to include names in transcripts from interviews, workshops or focus groups. Often it is sufficient to be able to relate specific data to certain types of user characteristic, such as age, gender or ethnicity. The basic underlying principle is that it should be impossible to identify any individual from the data.

Confirming the data

Sometimes the way in which we understand what users say is not what they meant. It is good practice to send a transcript of an interview or an account of a workshop to each user who participated and ask them to confirm the interpretation of the meeting. Often this process results in more and richer views being expressed, and it ensures that the resulting report truly reflects the views of the users who participated.

Ethics committees

All NHS trusts have a Local Research Ethics Committee that is bound by the advice of the Department of Health but not the General Medical Council. However, the vast majority of user involvement activities do not require the approval of Research Ethics Committees. Most user involvement is not research but service evaluation and development.

If you are unsure about whether you are doing 'research', ask yourself the following questions.

- Is the main purpose of the proposed user involvement programme to evaluate and improve local services?
- Are you planning to involve only users of your services?

If the answers are 'yes', you need not apply for approval from the Local Research Ethics Committee.

If you are unsure about your need to apply to an ethics committee, you could telephone them or your Research and Development department. There are approximately 250 Local Research Ethics Committees across the UK, which operate using different application forms, seek different information and meet at different times. You can find details of which ethics committee to apply to at www.corec.org.uk/LRECContacts.htm.

Reference

- Barley V, Daniel R *et al.* (1999) *Meeting the Needs of People With Cancer for Support and Self-Management: summary report.* Bristol Cancer Help Centre, Bristol.

Further reading

- Central Office for Research Ethics Committees; www.corec.org.uk
- Department of Health Research Governance; www.doh.gov.uk/research/rd3/nhsrandd/researchgovernance/govhome.htm
- World Medical Association Declaration of Helsinki (amended 2002) *Ethical Principles for Medical Research Involving Human Subjects;* www.wma.net/e/policy/b3.htm

Commission for Health Improvement guidelines on user involvement

**Patients and the public:
'NOTHING ABOUT US WITHOUT US'
A Patient and Public Strategy for the Commission
for Health Improvement**

The Commission for Health Improvement (CHI) is the independent authoritative voice on the state of the NHS. Our role is to help the NHS improve the quality of care provided to patients. We do this by reviewing patient care in every NHS organisation. We also conduct investigations where there has been a serious service failure and produce national studies on key health priorities.

The CHI has developed a strategy to define our work with patients and the public. Three key principles underpin our work.

- *Working for patients, service users, carers and the public*
  This means working on behalf of patients to ensure that they get the best quality care and treatment.
- *Working with patients, service users, carers and the public*
  This means involving patients and carers to ensure that they have a say in their care and treatment, and in the planning of local healthcare arrangements.
- *Working to patients, carers and the public*
  This means seeing how well the NHS serves its local community.

We shall use these principles as a guide to our work.

1 *Support a patient-centred NHS* — When we work with and assess NHS organisations, we will find out to what extent they are 'patient centred'. For example, we will:
  - look at the things that matter to patients
  - obtain patient and carer perspectives on what happens

- see whether patients, carers and the public have a say in things
- give people information on how good services are
- help organisations to do all of these things better.

2 *Use patient-centred methods*
When we work with and assess NHS organisations, we will use methods that are patient centred. For example, we will:
- involve patients and the public in our review teams and in developing the way in which we assess organisations
- use effective ways of obtaining the views of patients, carers and the public and community and voluntary organisations.

3 *Practise what we preach*
CHI will be patient centred. For example, we will:
- be open about what we do and the way we make decisions
- respond well to people who contact us
- communicate clearly what we do
- make specific efforts for people who do not speak English as a first language, who cannot read, or who have sensory impairments.

4 *Have the people and resources to do the work well*
CHI will have the capacity (the people, the internal systems and processes) to do this work properly. For example, we will:
- make sure that we have good systems to support all of the above
- support staff to take part in the work
- support patients, carers and the public in taking part in the work.

5 *Be socially inclusive*
We will make specific efforts to engage all sections of society in our work. For example, we will:
- build on the work we have done on ethnic diversity
- focus on people's individual needs
- focus on removing the barriers that prevent people receiving good care.

6 *Patient and public events*
Events were held during March 2002 to provide an opportunity for community and voluntary organisations to help CHI shape our work with patients and the public. Approximately 350 delegates shared ideas on how CHI can become more effective in this area. We have already taken steps on some of the points raised, such as improvements to CHI posters used in trusts and identifying more effective ways

of engaging local groups in CHI reviews. The findings from the conference and how we take forward the patient and public strategy will be available here shortly.

If you would like to contribute to share your experience – good and bad – at an NHS organisation that we are currently reviewing, please do call CHI on 0845 601 3012.

Commission for Health Improvement (2002) *'Nothing About Us Without Us': a patient and public strategy for the Commission for Health Improvement*; www.chi.nhs.uk/patients/index.shtml

Improving cancer services by involving service users: evaluation form

We are keen to evaluate the usefulness of this *Toolkit*. We would be grateful if you could complete the short evaluation form and return it to the Macmillan Project Officer for User Involvement, ASWCS, King Square House, King Square, Bristol BS2 8EE.

The evaluation form is also available on the ASWCS website, www.aswcs.nhs.uk.

1 What is your job title/role? _____

2 How did you hear about the *Toolkit*? _____
_____
_____

3 In what type of organisation has the *Toolkit* been used?
   Primary care trust   ☐   Cancer network   ☐
   Acute trust   ☐   Voluntary sector organisation   ☐
   Mental health trust   ☐   Partnership forum   ☐
   Hospice   ☐   Other (please specify)   ☐

4 How have you planned/are you planning to use this *Toolkit*?
_____
_____
_____

5 How was the *Toolkit* useful?
_____
_____

6 Was the *Toolkit* easy to use?
_____
_____

- Was it easy to find the information you were looking for?   Yes ☐   No ☐
- Did the layout of the *Toolkit* make it easy to use?   Yes ☐   No ☐
- Was it easy to use the tools included in the *Toolkit*?   Yes ☐   No ☐

7 How have you used the tools included in the *Toolkit* as part of a user involvement project?
_____
_____
_____

8 Do you have any suggestions on how the *Toolkit* can be improved?
_____
_____
_____

9 Do you have any other comments?
_____
_____
_____

Please return to ASWCS, FREEPOST (SWB1590), Bristol BS2 8ZZ

Many thanks for helping us by taking the time to complete this form.

PART 2

Tools and methods

A glossary of tools and methods for user involvement*

Strategies for user involvement in health services

Strategy	Degree of involvement	Key attributes
1 Publications, press releases and posters	Supports user involvement	Provide information on how users can participate. No requirement for dialogue
2 User information about service and treatment options	Supports user involvement	Printed and/or oral information presented in an accessible and understandable way. Explains treatment choices and likely outcomes, and outlines pathways for seeking answers to questions
3 Patient charters	Supports user involvement	Written definition of patient rights and guarantees specifying service conditions. Should provide pathways for complaints and possible redress if these conditions are not met
4 Staff development for user involvement	Supports user involvement	Job design, recruitment, orientation and training to inform and support user involvement
5 User-friendly administrative procedures	Supports user involvement	Review and adapt administrative communication with users to promote user involvement and partnerships
6 Volunteers	Supports user involvement	Unpaid workers who because of close contact with users often have the opportunity to obtain user feedback. Training, supervision and support are required from paid staff

*This is adapted based on our research from *Improving Health Services Through Consumer Participation. A resource guide for organisations*. Department of Health, Flinders University, and the South Australian Community Health Research Unit, Adelaide.

Strategy	Degree of involvement	Key attributes
7 Evaluation of services	Supports user involvement/ information seeking	Essential component of user involvement. Many methods. *See* Part 1, Section 5 for a detailed description
8 Participation in project groups	Can be information seeking or consultation	Organisation led to advise on specific issues and/or to guide a project. Time limited. May be used to demonstrate the value of user involvement to others
9 Research	Information seeking	Different models and methods. Most forms of research can incorporate aspects of user involvement
10 Surveys	Information seeking	Means of gathering information from users. Agenda set by organisations. Quantitative data
11 In-depth user interviews	Information seeking	Extended, semi-structured (usually) face-to-face interviews. Provide rich information from selected users. Useful for exploring particular issues and/or for specific population groups, but time consuming
12 Focus groups	Information seeking	Semi-structured interviews with 6–8 people lasting from 30 minutes to 2 hours. Participants are selected on the basis of who they are and what they can contribute to the discussion. Interactions between participants can help to explore issues in depth. Used for information collection on specific issues (not for decision making). Provides rich information, but may not be representative of all users
13 Submissions	Information seeking	Oral and written presentation of views. Can attract users who are organised and in a position to put in a submission. However, the less articulate/literate, those with non-English-speaking background and/or socially disadvantaged users may be excluded. May promote discussion
14 Delphi technique	Information seeking	Formal process using a series of mailed surveys to selected individuals. Relies on good literacy skills. Used for building consensus among users with conflicting views. Can also be used for exploring different perspectives. May be useful for particular groups of stakeholders on specific contentious issues

Strategy	Degree of involvement	Key attributes
15 Nominal group technique	Information seeking	Small-group process for reviewing options options and clarifying priorities in relation to a single issue. Does not generate rich data for exploring issues in depth, but can support decision making and allocating scarce resources, etc.
16 Suggestion boxes	Information seeking	Easy to implement, but limited for obtaining useful feedback. May attract negative and unhelpful comments. Only for use in conjunction with other strategies. Limited to those with literacy skills
17 Hotlines and phone-ins	Information seeking	Information gathering. Relies on publicity and on skilled staff or volunteers to answer phones. Attracts respondents, but is unrepresentative
18 Complaints heading	Information seeking/ consultation	Response to user feedback and complaints. Valuable resource because it is restricted to users who have identified a possible area for service improvement. Requires staff understanding of value of complaints. Unrepresentative of all dissatisfaction or potential complaints
19 Responding to user initiatives	Information seeking/ consultation	How your organisation/team responds to inquiries or requests initiated by users. Important to develop clear policies, processes and skills that are 'response-able'
20 Workshops	Information seeking/ consultation	Working meeting usually of 8–12 users, possible with providers to share information and to develop a joint approach to a specific issue. Participants have usually been selected on the basis of particular skills, knowledge or experience. Requires informed participants
21 User advocates/ consultants	Information seeking/ consultation, partnership	Healthcare organisation employee responsible for consulting with users and being an advocate on their behalf
22 Promotions and campaigns	Support user involvement, may include consultation and/or involvement	Ways to disseminate information. Can be innovative and creative and involve users, through consultation and partnership in planning and implementation

Strategy	Degree of involvement	Key attributes
23 Search conferences	Information seeking/ consultation	Meeting of 30–50 invited people. Investigates a subject/issue in a planned manner. May use discussion paper as a starter. Asks specific search question. Wide range of views canvassed, and discussion should lead to an answer
24 Public inquiries and hearings	Information seeking/ consultation	Instigated by organisations. Formal terms of reference. Receives public submissions (oral and written). Formal and possibly intimidating and likely to exclude views of socially disadvantaged users
25 Discussion papers	Information seeking/ consultation	Written presentation of information for discussion. May be used as precursor to public meetings or other discussion
26 Public meetings and forums	Information seeking/ consultation	Open meeting structured to canvass views and invite debate. Representatives nominated by user groups/associations. Open to public
27 Input into needs assessment process	Information seeking/ consultation	Cyclical planning process. Input may be requested by organisation using any of the information-seeking or consultation strategies listed here. If a permanent planning cycle, then can use standing committees with user representatives
28 Seminars and conferences	Information seeking/ consultation	Instigated by organisations to explore ideas/issues. May be restricted to those who can pay. Structured, formal presentations with informal or spontaneous input restricted to discussion. May be intimidating for some users
29 User councils and reference groups	Consultation	Structure and role defined by organisation. Composed of users who advise the organisation. Need to ensure that support for user representative is provided and links with appropriate constituency. Representatives need to have tenure long enough to learn to be useful, but not so long that they become part of the organisation. More than one user representative is needed
30 Policy round tables	Consultation	Invitations to structured discussion of policy items. Usually convened to advise on the development of specific policy

Strategy	Degree of involvement	Key attributes
31 User representatives on committees	Consultation	Need clear guidance on roles and the terms of reference. Provision of training and support. Promote representatives' links with specific constituency. A medium to long-term investment. Need more than one representative
32 Recruiting user representatives	Consultation	Need clear objectives for having user representatives. Identify and develop clear and effective processes for finding and selecting the types of users being sought
33 Consultative or advisory committees	Consultation	Usually up to about 15 members. To provide input on issues on the basis of expertise about an issue or relevant experience. Members can be appointed or elected. Usually limited term
34 Patient forums	Consultation	Patients invited to focus on an area/issue. Usually structured
35 User involvement policy	Supporting user involvement/ consultation/ partnership	User involvement policies provide an organisational approach to supporting and promoting user involvement. Policies guide the development of multiple strategies across the organisation to increase staff capacity as well as to foster and act on user involvement
36 Access policies and processes	Consultation	A formal process of structured involvement that is part of planning or resource allocation consultations, or may arise out of lack of use of services. Various consultation techniques may be used
37 User input into organisational or team policies	Consultation	Both formal and informal mechanisms. May include user representatives, management committees, planning groups, planning processes and policy development process
38 Facilitating mutual support groups	Supporting user involvement/ consultation/ therapeutic partnerships	Support to assist users who are to be involved. User groups may be consulted about service improvement. Clinicians can enter into partnership with groups as expert advisers

Strategy	Degree of involvement	Key attributes
39 Negotiation partnership	Consultation/ partnership	Users and providers work together to develop a written agreement by users and providers. Requires clarity of objectives and good communication skills
40 Networking	Consultation/ partnership	Informal relationship building with people who have common interests or goals. Will include building links to user organisations, advocacy groups and across different clinical and professional divides
41 Partnership of users and providers	Partnership	Structured cyclical planning process with specified role for users in shared decision making with providers. Process and outcomes are a shared responsibility. Usually the result of years of development of user involvement and a strong user focus and culture in the organisation
42 Community development	Partnership	Organic and flexible approach with a focus on process as well as outcomes. Scope for creative ways to facilitate involvement. Support and partnership with users about their own issues
43 Community control	Community control	Community elects board of directors. Management reports to board. Strong primary healthcare orientation with public health and social justice advocacy, but likely to involve conflict management

Methods and procedures

A: The nominal group technique

Stage 1: defining the question

It is important to structure the nominal group technique (NGT) process around an appropriate question. Participants should be asked to respond to a single question or statement rather than to complex, multiple questions. Questions such as 'What are the key issues to consider when involving users in service development?' or 'What changes may be needed to enhance user involvement in your area?' are suitable.

Stage 2: defining participants – who should be involved?

Careful selection of NGT participants is crucial. It is important to identify all of the groups of people who might have an interest in or a perspective on the issue that is being consulted about. In cancer services, these might include users from a number of different groups, ranging from those already 'involved' as members of voluntary-sector organisations to those who are not recognised as users. A number of different professional groups also need to be involved, depending on the question being asked.

Although the NGT can involve relatively small numbers of participants, it is important that these reflect the views of the wider constituents. It is also important to find a way of feeding back the results to the wider group (see discussion of the Delphi technique below).

It is also important to include participants from the range of population groups that are affected by the issue being considered. Factors such as gender, age, ethnicity and cancer type need to be considered. To some extent, participation rates may be influenced by structural factors. For example, the fact that women represent the majority of nurses will influence gender representation among this group. Ethnicity and socio-economic inequalities may also affect participation. It may be easier for professionals to involve articulate, educated users than other groups – difficulties of access and language may need to be overcome, requiring movement beyond conventional recruitment methods towards outreach and liaison with a wide number of groups and agencies. These difficulties intersect with aspects of the cancer experience that can also influence user participation. For example, differences in disease progression and survival rates may make it more difficult to include users with certain types of cancer, such as lung cancer, than those with others, including breast cancer. These issues present some difficult challenges, but the validity of the consensus development process is likely to be undermined if minority group perspectives are not included.

Stage 3: preparation

In order to help participants to prepare for the exercise, it is useful if prepara-tory materials are sent out in advance. These might include, if available, summaries of research evidence on the topic being discussed. Alternatively, relevant policy documents could be provided. Participants should be notified in advance of the topic for discussion, and they should be asked to prepare by making their own notes about it. When doing this, they should be asked to draw on a range of relevant sources of information, including both the research evidence (if provided) and their personal experience. It should be made clear that these are personal notes and do not have to be shared with the group, and that there will be time during the session to include new ideas that they had not thought of in advance. Participants should be given an outline of the procedure and this should explain the aims of the exercise, giving a schedule for the session so that they arrive with clear expectations.

Stage 4: group size and composition

Group size is a key factor to consider in consensus development. Groups with less than five participants may find it difficult to generate sufficient ideas and debate to analyse the problem. Larger groups can be difficult to manage and may not offer a very satisfying experience for participants. It is therefore recommended that groups include between 6 and 12 individuals. Large groups can be subdivided and parallel sessions held, although if this happens there needs to be a follow-up exercise to enable the results to be fed back to participants.

The make-up of the groups can affect the result of any consensus develop-ment exercise. For example, groups that consist of diverse individuals may be less likely to reach a consensus than groups composed of individuals from similar backgrounds. The make-up of the groups will depend on the aim of the exercise. If this is to explore perspectives and address issues of uncertainty, then there may be good reasons for having diverse groups. On the other hand, if the aim is to reach group consensus about key issues, then membership can be restricted to members of the same profession or user group, provided that the results are not assumed to be valid for other groups.

Stage 5: the group discussion

The group discussion takes about two hours and requires one, or prefer-ably two, skilled facilitators. In addition, it is useful for an observer to be present to make notes about the process for evaluation purposes. A check-list of resources needed for the session is provided below.

The NGT involves a structured group discussion organised into three phases.

Phase 1: silent generation of ideas

During this stage, participants reflect on their preparation notes and write down any further responses to the question being discussed.

Phase 2: round robin recording of ideas

During this stage, each participant in turn states one idea, which is written on a flipchart or board that is visible to all participants. At this stage there is no discussion of the ideas. This is to allow each participant a say and to make sure that all of the ideas are recorded. Participants should be reminded that they are not required to contribute during any round, and that if they pass during one round they will not forfeit their right to contribute during the next round. New ideas that had not been thought of during the preparation stage are likely to emerge, and these should be recorded. However, participants should be discouraged from offering ideas that simply repeat a contribution that has already been made.

Phase 3: discussion and clarification

Once the round robin is complete, there follows a discussion of each idea in turn. During this stage it should be made clear that the individuals who contributed the idea are not responsible for elaborating it, but rather the aim of the discussion is to clarify a shared meaning among the group for each statement. Participants may also debate the relative importance of each idea, proposing arguments in agreement or disagreement with it. During this stage, ideas that are similar to each other may be combined, but no statements should be deleted.

Phase 4: scoring and ranking

During this stage, participants are asked to rank or rate the items. This can be done in a number of ways. For example, each participant can be asked to identify the ten most important items from the list, and these can be combined to form the group's top ten statements. Alternatively, participants can be asked to give each item a numerical score, and the group ranking can be based on calculation of mean scores. A combination of both of these methods can also be used. This involves a ranking exercise followed by scoring of the top ten items. An example of this scoring method is provided in the NGT case study below. Examples of participants' and facilitators' score sheets are provided in Part 2, Section 3B.

Stage 6: evaluation

It is important to evaluate the procedure. Ideally, this should involve evaluation of both process and outcomes. Feedback from participants about their experiences of the process should be sought, using debriefing or other methods such as a simple, confidential and anonymous questionnaire. However, care is needed to ensure that this does not prove burdensome for participants. Qualitative methods are likely to be useful for evaluation – qualitative data can be collected by an observer if one is present during the NGT sessions. It is also important to compare NGT outcomes with outcomes achieved by other means in order to evaluate the benefits of the process.

B: A Delphi survey

Stage 1: preparation

This technique involves a series of questionnaires, each building on the results of the last one. The first stage involves individuals being asked to respond to a broad question, and each subsequent questionnaire is designed in the light of previous responses. It is important that the first questionnaire reflects the views of participants. The technique is often modified by using the NGT as a method of initial questionnaire development. In this way the NGT can be used to elicit responses to a question or prompt and the result can be incorporated into a Delphi questionnaire that is then distributed to a larger number of people. An example of a stage-one Delphi questionnaire developed using this method is provided in Part 2, Section 3C.

Stage 2: selecting participants

The selection of participants is a key issue. It is important that participants reflect the full range of groups and constituencies that might be affected by the issue. With regard to user involvement, this may include patients, carers and members of voluntary organisations as well as professionals. It is also important to consider the social and demographic characteristics of participants – particular efforts may be needed to recruit 'hard-to-reach' and minority groups.

Differences in responses between groups need to be considered. Some groups may be more willing to respond or may be more familiar with questionnaires and surveys, and this might affect the results. The questionnaires should therefore be designed in a way that makes them accessible to a wide range of people. The use of the NGT as a method of questionnaire development can help in this respect, as the elements within the questionnaire can be written to reflect participants' own language and responses to the initial prompt.

Stage 3: questionnaire rounds

The Delphi technique involves more than one questionnaire round. Participants are usually sent feedback from the first questionnaire in which both individual and group results are presented. This allows individuals to reflect on their views in relation to the group judgement. Subsequent feedback and questionnaires allow additional opportunities for reflection and re-ranking. The process stops either when consensus has been approached or when the number of responses diminishes beyond a useful point.

Stage 4: analysing the results

There are many different ways of analysing the results of a Delphi process. These are discussed in Further reading on page 44, and it is worth bearing in mind that the technique does depend on some knowledge of statistical data collection and analysis. A key issue is the definition of consensus. This can be defined in different ways, but difficulties can result if the threshold is either too high or too low. It is also important to note that consensus does not necessarily indicate the 'correct' position – majority views can reflect the fact that most people are mistaken or misinformed!

Stage 5: dissemination

Dissemination is a key issue. Consensus development can produce useful outputs, but often the real benefits relate to the process, which can be educational for participants and can be extended at the dissemination stage. Furthermore, it is important that the results of consensus development are implemented, and the dissemination process can help with this.

Stage 6: evaluation

It is important to evaluate the procedure. Ideally, this should involve evaluation of both process and outcomes. Feedback from participants about their experiences of the process can be sought using questionnaires.

C: A user involvement mapping questionnaire

Stage 1: who are your respondents?

The first thing you need to consider is who you want to obtain information from. Who is going to be filling in your questionnaire? You need to consider the different types of groups and organisations that you may wish to contact (sometimes voluntary organisations are as important as NHS organisations). You also need to think about which individuals within the organisation should know about or have responsibility for user involvement. Sending a questionnaire to someone who has nothing to do with user involvement will result in a form that is left blank or not returned. You need to put together a list of your intended respondents. If you are planning to post your questionnaire, you also need to have the correct postal address and titles. This list is your sample, and it is these people who you are going to ask to fill in your questionnaire.

Stage 2: writing your questionnaire

It is important that you do not start from scratch. There are many questionnaires that have been used extensively and are well validated (we have included some in Section 3). This is another case where *assisted wheel reinvention* is essential. Read some of the literature on user involvement and think carefully about what aspects of user involvement you are interested in. For instance, it may be that you want to focus on how users have been part of service evaluation. Such a focus must shape the type of questions you want to ask.

You want to include some questions about who is filling in your questionnaire. Sometimes the person to whom you send a questionnaire passes it on to someone else to fill in. It is probably a good idea to ask for information about job title and user involvement responsibilities. This may be important if you are trying to build up a network of people with expertise and experience of user involvement.

It is probably a good idea to include both closed questions (questions that have fixed answers) and open questions (questions that ask people to write a short answer). However, you need to think about how you are going to analyse the completed questionnaires when they are returned.

Examples of open and closed questions

- If you had a larger budget for user involvement activities, what would you spend it on? (open question)

- What is the budget for user involvement activities in your organisation, unit or department? (closed question)

    Under £100   £101–500   £501–£1000   Over £1000

It is important that you leave enough space for people to answer open questions, and that the responses you provide for closed questions are mutually exclusive and cover the entire potential set of possible responses (they are exhaustive).

Sometimes you may be interested in people's opinions or personal views, but want to capture them in a way that allows you to compare them. It may be useful to use Likert-scale questions. This type of question asks people to evaluate a statement in terms of the extent to which they agree or disagree with it.

Example of question using a Likert scale

- Users' views can best be incorporated through shared decision making with managers and clinicians.

    Agree strongly   Agree   Neither agree nor disagree
        Disagree   Disagree strongly

As well as your questionnaire, you need to write a covering letter explaining briefly what you are doing and why, and emphasising how important it is that as many people respond as possible. It may be worth stating in the letter that you are very interested in their responses, and you should include a deadline for completing the questionnaire (allow a minimum of two weeks). *See* page 168.

Stage 3: piloting your questionnaire

After you have drafted the questions for your questionnaire and thought about the layout and presentation of your survey, it is important to see how other people understand it. This piloting process involves identifying a number of people (at least ten) who are like those whom you want to complete your survey, and asking them to try to fill in the questionnaire. It is probably also a good idea not to ask people who are part of the sample from whom you want to collect information.

After your pilot group has read the covering letter and filled in the questionnaire, ask to go through it with them and talk about the different questions. The main aim of this stage is to understand which questions are difficult to understand and how to reword them to make them clearer. It also provides an opportunity to check that questions are understood in the same way by the respondents. The comments from the pilot respondents need to be integrated into the covering letter and questionnaire.

Stage 4: administering your questionnaire

Now you have finalised your covering letter and questionnaire (stage 3) it is time to distribute it to your respondents. Address envelopes and enclose the questionnaire, a copy of the covering letter that you have signed (it makes a difference if you sign them individually) and a return envelope. Make sure that you put an ID number on each questionnaire and note to whom it was posted, as it is important to keep track of those individuals who have not responded so that you can send them a reminder letter.

If you are asking people to return their completed questionnaires by hand that is fine, but if you want to post the questionnaires you should make sure that you have included the correct postage on the reply envelope. It is worth checking to see whether your organisation has a FREEPOST number, as this usually works out a lot cheaper than individual stamps. If you are sending a large number of questionnaires or are planning to conduct a number of surveys, you may want to find out whether obtaining your own FREEPOST number would be worthwhile.

After the deadline you included in your covering letter for completing the questionnaire has passed, you should send out a reminder letter. This should emphasise the importance of each individual response and suggest that the respondent may have misplaced the questionnaire. Include with the reminder letter another copy of the questionnaire (with another ID number).

Stage 5: looking at the responses – coding and analysing your data

Once the questionnaires have been returned you will begin to record the information they contain in a standard way (this is called *coding*). If you are only surveying a few people (less than 20), it may be best to use a word processor or spreadsheet. It is probably worth copying all of the different responses from open questions on to a word-processing file and thinking about particular themes and issues that emerge. Qualitative analysis (i.e. the analysis of written or spoken data) is also a specialist skill, and it may be worth getting some advice about this.

The basic idea behind coding and analysis is to identify themes and patterns that emerge from the questionnaires when you have recorded them in a standardised way that allows comparison between questionnaires. For more sophisticated types of analysis (e.g. looking at how age, gender and role relate to the types of responses provided) you will need to do more specialised quantitative and statistical analysis. If you are looking for quantitative information and statistical findings, you will need to obtain specialist advice about how to code and analyse your data.

The findings from your mapping exercise are intended to form a baseline indication of the level of user involvement that is occurring in a particular set of organisations. It is important that you undertake the analysis appropriately, as the baseline you are establishing will be what you measure against to monitor change (hopefully improvement) in the knowledge, extent and type of user involvement that is occurring.

Stage 6: evaluating your mapping exercise

It is important that you look at the way in which your questionnaire was responded to. You want to be able to make a general statement about the level and knowledge of user involvement among the organisations that you surveyed (i.e. establish a baseline measurement). To be able to demonstrate that your findings are valid, you need to show what proportion of the people you sent questionnaires actually completed and returned them (the response rate).

You also need to look at the individuals who did not return a questionnaire. The key issue you want to check is whether there appear to be patterns among those who did not return the questionnaire. That is, did less than 50% of each category of respondents complete and return a questionnaire? You need to consider what are the most relevant categories for your exercise, but they might include gender, job title and type of work setting.

Stage 7: evaluation – was your mapping exercise successful?

There are a number of ways to evaluate how well your mapping exercise has proceeded. The first is to look at who responded to the questionnaire and who did not. Are there identifiable patterns among those who did not complete a questionnaire? For instance, did people from only one particular part of the organisation fill in and return the questionnaire? Or perhaps only men completed your survey.

A second way to think about how well the mapping exercise has gone is to look at how completely the questionnaires were filled in. That is, were there some questions that tended to be left blank or that people seemed to answer in a strange way (e.g. by ticking more than one box)?

Both of these are measures of how complete your information is and how representative it is of the group of people you chose to include in your mapping exercise. A final way in which you could think about evaluating how the exercise went is to consider the user involvement activities that you know are going on, and see whether they are included in the responses you have received. If they are not, then you need to think about why they were not captured with the questionnaire you were using.

D: Running a focus group

Stage 1: define the purpose of your focus group

Stating a clear aim for your focus group will help you to develop appropriate questions, identify the relevant participants and obtain the information you need from them.

Stage 2: identify participants

Who do you want to involve in the focus group? Is it just patients, or do you want to involve carers, healthcare staff, referring agencies, the public, etc.? Once you have defined the population from which you want to draw your participants, decide how many participants you need. As a rough guide, each focus group should involve six to ten people. Invite twice the number you need to allow for those who do not reply, have moved away, etc. Which individuals are you going to invite to take part?

Obtain contact details for those people you are going to invite. Keeping this information on a computer database such as Microsoft Access can save a lot of time in the long term, as you can then send out invitations (called a Mail Merge) and keep a record of responses.

Stage 3: recruit a facilitator

Effective facilitation is essential for a good focus group. This involves good communication skills and an awareness of group dynamics. If possible this person should be neutral (i.e. not an employee of your organisation) and, if your budget will allow for it, a professional facilitator is the preferred option.

Stage 4: send out invitations

Include a clear description of your project and some background reading material. This will increase the response rate and prepare participants for the focus group discussion.

Stage 5: generate and develop questions

Having a few prepared questions will help to focus discussions on the issues that you want to consider. Open-ended questions work best in terms of encouraging group discussion. Reading background literature that is related to your topic should help you to develop these questions. An in-depth interview with one of your potential participants is another way of generating a list of questions. These can then be merged to produce three or four questions as a structure for the focus group. Test out your final list of questions on a group of people who will not take part in the study (e.g. a group of colleagues).

Stage 6: prepare a script

Even experienced facilitators find that a script contributes to the smooth running of a focus group. It can be divided into three sections, namely an introduction (welcoming participants and describing the purpose of the group and how a focus group works), questions (using the questions you developed to structure discussions) and close (thanking participants and explaining how their input will be used).

Stage 7: choose a venue

A comfortable room helps to put participants at ease. Factors to consider include the following. Is it a neutral setting? Is it the right size for the number of participants? Is it easily accessible in terms of public transport, parking, disabled access, etc.? Is the seating arrangement appropriate?

Stage 8: convene the focus group

Make sure that you have all of the materials in the checklist above available. Be there early to welcome participants as they arrive. If you are recording the session, remember to test your equipment beforehand.

Stage 9: analyse the data

Either using qualitative data-analysis software (e.g. Atlas.ti) or by hand, analyse the focus group transcripts and note any patterns, trends, repeated phrases, etc.

Stage 10: evaluation (how do you know whether what you have done is any good?)

Looking at the aims you set for the focus group(s), do the results tell you what you wanted to know? Will you be able to use the information that you have gathered to improve services? After using any method of documenting service user experiences, it is also important to give participants the opportunity to say how it was for them. A range of methods can be used for this, including feedback forms, questionnaires and debriefing interviews.

Stage 11: dissemination

It is important to tell people what you found. This includes writing up the project and providing feedback to participants. (For more information, *see* Part 1, Section 8 on implementation and dissemination.)

E: Interviews

Stage 1: define the aim of your interviews

Be clear about what information you are looking for. This can help you to choose what types of interviews to use. The more depth of information you require, the less structured your interviews will need to be.

Stage 2: identify potential participants

Whose views do you want to collect? Is it just those of patients, or do you want to include carers, healthcare staff, referring agencies or the general public? Once you have defined the group from which you want to draw your participants, decide how many participants you need. Bear in mind that interviews are very time-consuming to conduct and analyse. Invite twice the number you need to allow for those who do not reply or who have moved away. Assuming that you do not have time to interview everyone, how will you decide who to invite? There are various ways of selecting a sample (*see* page 24 on sampling procedures for more information).

Stage 3: obtain contact details

You will need to obtain the names and addresses of the people you want to invite to take part. Keeping this information on a computer database such as Microsoft Access can save a lot of time in the long term, as you can then send out invitations (called a Mail Merge) and keep a record of responses.

Stage 4: send out invitations

Include a clear description of your project and some background reading material. This can increase the number of people who are willing to take part, as well as helping to prepare participants for the interviews.

Stage 5: develop an interview schedule

You need an interview schedule to make sure that you cover all of the topics you need to and that you ask all of your participants the same questions. For structured interviews you will need a comprehensive list of all the questions you plan to ask. Less structured interviews require fewer questions in order to cover general subject areas. The aim of these questions is to prompt the participants to give you the information that you need. Some people will be more forthcoming than others, so it is worth having some supplementary questions in case the answers to your main questions do not tell you what you need to know. Reading the background literature related to your topic should help you to develop these questions. You could also conduct a pilot interview with one person in order to develop ideas.

Stage 6: prepare a script

When conducting interviews it is a good idea to follow a common structure. This could include introducing yourself, explaining the project aims, emphasising confidentiality, thanking participants for taking part and explaining how their interviews will be used. The best way to achieve this is to prepare a script covering these main areas.

Stage 7: choose a location

Participants should ideally be offered a choice of interview location. Their own home is often the preferred option, and it provides a more relaxed atmosphere. However, some participants may prefer to come to your organisation's offices or to a neutral venue, such as a café or a room in the premises of a local community organisation. It is also important to conduct interviews at a convenient time for the participants in order to fit in with their lifestyles. It is standard practice to offer to pay participants for travel costs and any other expenses. Some people also feel it is appropriate to offer some form of payment for participants' time. Check whether your organisation has any guidelines on this.

Stage 8: carry out the interviews

If you are taping the interviews, make sure that you have an adequate supply of tapes and batteries. Being interviewed can raise emotional issues for participants, so it is important to make sure that support is available for those who require it. This could include the contact details for support organisations such as CancerBACUP. It can also be an emotional experience for the researcher who is conducting the interview, so a system for accessing support should be clearly identified.

Stage 9: analyse the data

Once they have been transcribed, interviews can be analysed either by computer using qualitative data-analysis software (e.g. Atlas.ti) or by hand. The basic aim of content analysis is to identify overall themes and note any quotes which might support them. Validate your work by asking someone else to analyse some of the interviews and comparing your findings.

Stage 10: evaluation (how do you know whether what you have done is any good?)

Did you find out what you set out to discover? Has this information been useful in terms of evaluating or developing services? How was the experience for those who took part? These are some of the questions that can form part of your evaluation process.

Stage 11: dissemination

Now that you have completed a user involvement initiative, it is important to tell people about it. For more information on how to do this, *see* Part 1, Section 8 on implementation and dissemination.

F: Setting up a website

Stage 1: deciding on the purpose of the website

You need to decide what your reasons are for having a website. Which groups may find this website useful? What type of information would they need on this website? Consultation with health professionals or service users will ensure that this site is of relevance to them.

Stage 2: website design

The starting point of your website is what is called a *home page*. It is important that your home page is not overloaded with information. You may want to have a brief overview of your project. You should also make clear links to the other pages of your website. Useful links could include ways in which service users can be included, a project newsletter (if available), a 'what's new in this project' page, and a comments section. Do remember to include a contact email address on your home page.

You should try to be considerate and not use too many graphics, as not everyone has access to a high-speed modem. You need to check any institutional guidelines or regulations on how your web page should appear. For example, the NHS has produced explicit guidelines on how to develop a web page.

Stage 3: getting the site online

Once you have prepared a website you will need to publish it on the Web. For this you will need to find a host for your website. There are two options here. Your organisation may have a local area network (LAN) that can host your site. Alternatively, you may need a commercial Internet service provider (ISP) to maintain your site.

Stage 4: making it happen

Once your website is online, you may also consider how you are going to publicise the site. The use of local media can be a good starting point. Do make sure that your website is registered with different search engines such as Google or Yahoo. Further information on how you can submit your website to the Google search engine can be found at http://dmoz.org/ add.html. It is also important to provide an opportunity for feedback.

Stage 5: updating your website

Do not forget to update your website regularly. By making regular updates you can ensure that people will visit your website again!

G: Developing a newsletter

Stage 1: define the purpose of the newsletter

The format and language of the newsletter will depend on your audience. Health professionals may want something different to what service users might find interesting. You may want to target both audiences, in which case you may need to clearly signpost the different sections of the newsletter aimed at different groups. A table of contents summarising what is included on the subsequent pages can be useful. Consulting service users can give you an idea of what they would expect from a newsletter.

Stage 2: focus on the logistics of this exercise

You need to spend some time thinking about the format of the newsletter. For example, you must decide on the number of pages per issue and how often it is going to be published. You will also need to decide how many copies of the newsletter you will need. You may also consider producing an electronic version of the newsletter. Your overall budget may determine your decisions at this stage.

Stage 3: print your newsletter

Once you have drafted the newsletter, it is a good idea to seek some assistance with regard to the layout and presentation style. You may need some help with plain English. You can always check whether your organisation has a press officer, as a chat with them is always useful. The publisher can assist you with the layout, although it is advisable to format your draft using desktop publishing software (e.g. Microsoft Publisher or Quark).

Stage 4: distribute your newsletter

Your newsletter is now ready to be distributed. Make sure that you have included contact details so that people can contact you if necessary.

Stage 5: obtain some feedback

It is important to find out what people think of your efforts. Make sure that there is a system for feedback of comments and suggestions, and use these when designing your next edition. You might even ask your readers to make their own contributions.

H: Running a workshop

Stage 1: define the purpose of the workshop

It is important to be clear about your aims and how you plan to achieve them. Sometimes it is best to devise smaller-scale activities as a lead-in to the main activity.

Stage 2: identify potential participants – who do you want to take part in the workshop?

It could be just service users, or you might want to include some health-care professionals. There are no limits on numbers, but you might want to consider breaking up into smaller groups for activity-based sessions.

Stage 3: send out invitations

Explain what you plan to do and what you hope to achieve. You might want to send participants some background information on workshops in general and the issue(s) you are dealing with in particular, as well as the obvious details such as how to get there. Don't forget to ask about people's special needs in terms of hearing, sight, language, mobility and diet.

Stage 4: collect information in advance

It can be useful to collect ideas from participants in advance. For example, collating a list of the problems that people experience when using services can save time on the day.

Stage 5: structure the workshop

Break the time up into periods of about an hour, separated by breaks for refreshments. After an introductory session you might want to divide into smaller groups. Start each session with a brief description of what you hope to achieve and how you plan to do it. This may involve presentations, handouts or other documents. Give clear instructions for any tasks that you want participants to perform.

Stage 6: consider what materials you will need

Activities often require a range of equipment. Make sure that you have the necessary information and materials.

Stage 7: run the group

It is important to establish good communication between participants. Introductions and icebreakers are useful ways of putting people at ease. Everyone should be clear about the aims of the workshop. Describe the structure of the day as well as what will happen to the information produced. Each subgroup will want to report back to the larger group. This is an essential part of the workshop, but make sure that presentations are not too long, and keep to a common format.

Stage 8: reviewing the workshop

There is often a need to pull together what has been learnt from each subgroup and put it into some meaningful format. This can be done by a facilitator or by having a closing round during which each person states briefly what they feel has been achieved.

Stage 9: planning a course of action

In order to maintain the momentum which a workshop has generated, it is often best to convert the results into a plan of action.

Stage 10: evaluation

It is important to evaluate the effectiveness of a workshop, particularly if you are planning to run one again. Lessons can be learned in terms of how it was for the participants, the performance of facilitators, the structure of the day and the usefulness of the outcomes. Feedback sheets are a useful evaluation tool. These could include rating scales for different aspects of the workshop (e.g. content, activities, facilities, facilitation).

I: A user involvement training programme

Promoting Best Practice in User Involvement (PBPUI)

From our experience with the Interprofessional Cancer Education (IPCE) project, we had identified that health professionals needed several things. First, they needed to understand what was meant by the terms 'users' and 'user involvement' and to be able to explore safely a range of ways in which users might be involved and their views elicited so that they could select an appropriate method for their team or specialty. This is because there is no 'one size fits all' for user involvement in cancer services. Some professionals are dealing with a client group that is generally diagnosed early in their condition, such as breast cancer, but where there is extreme anxiety and an issue over 'false positives' in screening. Others are dealing with patients who are diagnosed at a stage when their condition is virtually untreatable and they are forced to make decisions about 'end-of-life' care.

Second, we had identified that professionals usually needed some 'hand-holding' along the way from a professional colleague with experience of user involvement. The role of this person was to act as a mentor and adviser to the teams. This role was needed because of the lack of confidence in the teams, and the tendency for senior members, such as doctors, to hand over responsibility for user involvement to their nursing colleagues without much in the way of practical support or encouragement. In the case of the IPCE project, the role of the mentor was taken on by the project facilitator. In the case of the PBPUI project it was provided by individuals who had previously been identified as having experience in user involvement, and who had been canvassed to elicit their active participation.

Third, we provided a small element of resources (i.e. funding) for each of the teams to access to help them to carry out their plans. This was not a large sum (in the range of £500), but it 'oiled the wheels' in that it could be used for things such as printing and distributing a questionnaire, providing refreshments and travel expenses for a meeting involving patients, or developing a patient information leaflet. The fact that this was helpful suggests that the allocation of a budget for user involvement, which is available to teams on the ground and under their control, is a helpful component of developing proactive user involvement. Teams within the IPCE project did not have this financial component, but they did have the benefit of being part of a larger project with a certain element of status for the organisation and individuals involved, and the reward (at least for some) of academic credit.

The educational process

An important element of the educational process that needs to be emphasised at the outset was that it was a co-operative venture between the network management and the local higher education provider, namely the University of the West of England. Different organisations bring with them different skills and qualities, and in this instance key components of success were that we drew together expertise in user involvement from the university (in terms of a lecturer who had recognised skills) and a senior manager in the network. The latter had direct contact with the teams and also had responsibility for accreditation. Thus she was aware that teams were going to need to demonstrate how they had worked with users, and encourage them to take advantage of this opportunity for support. Her wide links across the network also enabled her to identify individuals who might be able to provide mentorship support, and to invite them to participate. A final member of the team, whose main work was in the cancer voluntary sector, provided additional expertise and encouragement, and perhaps had more flexibility within her role to enable her to provide additional liaison between the network and the university. Neither the university nor the network could have achieved the educational initiative without this type of collaboration.

Both projects (IPCE and PBPUI) took place over approximately an academic year. For general purposes, the model was similar, but the PBPUI is described below because it is most suitable for general use where academic credit is not desired, necessary or available. In both the IPCE project and the PBPUI it was teams, rather than individuals, which were invited to participate. Of most relevance to others who are trying to institute the same process, the way in which teams are selected should to some extent reflect the organisational structure on the ground. In the case of the local network, the initiative was aimed at the multidisciplinary teams created around different cancer specialties. We also recognised that any process of change requires senior members of the team to be 'on board', even if at the end of the day it is others who will actually carry out the work. To this end, we started the process by inviting the teams to an introductory workshop (stage 1), and we encouraged senior members to attend. At the workshop, participants were provided with clear but detailed instructions on how the educational initiative would be carried out, and the process of starting to involve users was described in simple steps. Teams were also introduced to those individuals who would act as mentors during the process.

In total there were five stages to the programme, including the workshop described above. In stage 2, participants audited what was going on already, and identified one simple issue on which they would like to work. Consequently, the process we were encouraging was the same as or similar to the Plan–Do–Study–Act (PDSA) quality approach that was being used in the Cancer Collaboratives and other Department of Health initiatives.

Thus we hoped that participating teams and individuals would begin to see how these issues might be linked. Teams had about ten weeks to carry out this task (stage 2).

In September, stage 3 took place. This was another workshop that lasted a whole day, so that the teams could feed back 'where they were at', tell us about their issues, and plan what they wanted to do over the next six months. They brought a range of issues, from carrying forward a piece of work that had started well and then got stuck 'on a shelf', to quite a large-scale survey of communication between professionals and how this affected users. We employed the same university facilitator to run the day and provide a theoretical and practical framework. The mentors were also invited to attend.

Groups were then given approximately six months to complete their projects (stage 4), during which time they were encouraged and supported by their mentors, who in turn were supported by members of the group running the initiative. This was not intended to be heavy 'hands-on' facilitation, but rather support, encouragement, advice and prompts to action so that teams could conduct their projects. An essential component of this stage was that the teams were actively involved and worked with users in some way.

The final stage of the project (stage 5) was a concluding workshop in which groups were asked to demonstrate what they had been doing in the form of a simple presentation or poster. We suggested that the teams should invite one or two users to come with them to the presentation. In the event, the final presentation workshop was attended by managers from the teams' organisation and others with an interest in user involvement. Although this had seemed daunting, the process of producing a poster or presentation and describing how their project had developed proved extremely rewarding for the teams involved, and the posters gave them something which they could present in other arenas.

The result of the educational initiatives (both the PBPUI described above and the IPCE) was that the multidisciplinary teams involved were assisted in involving their users in addressing some aspect of service development. The most striking aspects of the evaluations of the programmes were first that the teams so profoundly required this type of structured facilitation to give them sufficient confidence to engage with users, and secondly, that they found the experience so deeply satisfying. One of the IPCE team members commented as follows:

> The thing that I learnt very much was that learning by practice and relating theory, although I learnt this at university, seeing it in action was very beneficial because it does work, because these lessons I'll carry forever now. I've learnt something that won't be taken away.

> (Team member, IPCE project)

On the following pages we present the Agenda for the Introductory Meeting of the IPCE project together with the Information Sheet that was distributed to participants.

Site-Specific Group User Involvement Training Project

Introductory Meeting, 10.30–12.30, Wednesday 28 June

University of the West of England, Glenside Campus

Programme

Time	Activity	Speaker/facilitator
10.00	Arrival and coffee	
10.30	Introductions and overall outline of the project	Project Manager, ASWCS Facilitator, ASWCS/ University of the West of England
11.00	Learning to work with users	Lecturer and Specialist in Consumer Involvement, Faculty of Health and Social Care, University of the West of England
11.30	Taking the project to multidisciplinary teams – the practicalities and support, forward planning	Small-group work with two facilitators
12.15	Feedback and discussion	All
12.30–13.00	Close and sandwich lunch	

Site-Specific Group User Involvement Training Project

Your Questions Answered!

Introduction

It is increasingly evident that to involve users in the development of services means that these services are more appropriate and accessible to those who use them. In many cases, this also means that the environments in which health professionals have to work become less stressful and more rewarding. In addition, it is likely that being able to demonstrate that users have been appropriately consulted will soon form part of the accreditation process. Avon, Somerset and Wiltshire Cancer Services have been fortunate to acquire funding to provide some training and support for *site specialist groups* (SSGs) and their associated *multidisciplinary teams* (MDTs) to help them to work out the best ways of working with their users.

Why is the training based around SSGs and MDTS?

It can be difficult to know how best to involve users, particularly when different types of cancer have such different disease trajectories. Different tumour sites will have different implications for ease or difficulty of communication, and issues of gender or social class may bring their own specific needs. There is no one 'right' way. However, people working in similar areas may have similar problems, and may be able to share ideas and concerns or give each other support and help. For this reason, we have focused the project on the SSGs and their associated MDTs.

Not more work! What do we have to do *now*?

We have tried to make this project really simple and achievable. It will last from July 2000 to March 2001, and will have five stages.

Stage 1: introductory workshop (28 June 2000) for SSG representatives

- We introduce you to the project and give you the opportunity to discuss how you want to take the project forward.
- We introduce each SSG/MDT representative to a colleague with experience of user involvement, who will provide some ongoing support and encouragement for those undertaking the project (each of these 'mentors' will have only one or two SSGs to support).

- We provide a checklist/framework for undertaking a simple 'audit' of any ways in which your MDT currently involves users in developing services.

Stage 2: finding out what is happening now (July to September 2000)

Each SSG/MDT conducts a simple audit, using the checklist or framework provided to ascertain the extent to which the views of users are currently sought, either formally or informally, and the extent to which this information is fed into any processes of staff development, training or service provision. Each MDT will be asked to identify *one* simple issue on which they would like to work.

Stage 3: MDT User Involvement Workshop (20 September 2000)

This workshop will last for a whole day, and should be attended by at least two members from each participating MDT. It will provide an opportunity to:

- feed back and compare findings of the audit/checklist undertaken over the summer, and discuss the issues that this has raised in the different areas
- learn about some ways in which user involvement has been tackled, examples of good practice and resources available (we will provide a simple resource pack)
- using the 'PDSA' model, discuss possible ways of involving users to help to address the issue that each group has raised
- develop a simple action plan.

Stage 4: involving users – getting to grips with the reality (September 2000 to March 2001)

- During this stage, each participating MDT will take forward the issue they have previously identified, making a specific effort to directly seek the views of users and/or supporters in their project.
- To help them to do this, they can continue to draw on the support of their 'mentor' – not always through 'meetings', but also by email and telephone support.
- Each group will have access to a small amount of funding (£250) from ASWCS to help them to carry this out. This is to cover such items as paying user expenses, funding 'hospitality' (e.g. sandwiches for a discussion group), or contributing to the cost of an educational visit to a unit that is doing similar work. Each group is entitled to a similar amount.

- Each group will develop a simple presentation or poster, by means of which they can demonstrate their work to others.

Stage 5: Feedback workshop (March 2001)

This workshop will provide an opportunity to:

- feed back and share information about projects undertaken by different MDTs
- reflect on the issues raised by the work of the past six months
- identify any areas of work to take forward.

We anticipate that, at this workshop, MDTs will feel confident enough to bring with them one or two users (or supporters) who have helped them with their project.

Final comments

These workshops are free to participants, and will be suitable for CME and PREP requirements.

Research tools validated during the project

A: Questionnaire for mapping user involvement

Below is the text used on the covering letter accompanying the mapping user involvement questionnaire. The intent of the letter is to explain the main aims of the research and encourage respondents to complete and return the questionnaire. The questionnaire itself begins on the next page.

This questionnaire asks you to tell us about any NHS user involvement activity that your voluntary organisation or support group is (or has been) part of. User involvement may consist of asking patients and carers for their views on the service, or asking them to help make decisions about new developments. However, there are many different interpretations of the term 'user involvement', and we are interested to see what it means to you in your organisation. This will complement the information we have already collected from NHS organisations. Please answer the following sets of questions from the perspective of *your group or organisation*.

Even if you feel that your organisation does not participate in user involvement at present, we would be grateful if you would complete Section 1 and read through the whole questionnaire to see whether any questions apply to your organisation. In the final section there is also an opportunity for you to outline any experience you have with involving users in your own organisation or group, and any future plans you may have in this area.

Section 1: Your details

First, please give us some basic background information about you and your organisation.

1 What is your name?

2 How did you receive this questionnaire?

 ☐ Posted to me directly

 ☐ Passed to me by

3 What is the name of your voluntary organisation?

 Please give a brief description of the type of organisation or group, and enclose any relevant leaflets.

4 How long have you worked/been involved with this organisation?
 years   months

Section 2: Your organisation's involvement in NHS services

The next set of questions asks for details of any involvement your organisation or group has had with NHS services. Please read through all of the questions to see which of them you can answer. Don't worry, however, if they do not apply to your particular group or organisation.

1 How would your organisation define 'users' of NHS cancer services?

2 What experience, if any, has your organisation had in participating in NHS user involvement activities? (please give details)

3 Who in your organisation is responsible for responding to requests for help with NHS user involvement activities, if anyone?
  Name:
  Job title:
  Contact telephone no.:

4 What characteristics make the most effective involved user (e.g. age, cancer type)?

5 For your group or organisation, what is the purpose of user involvement in NHS cancer services? (In other words, why should you do it?)

6 What training, if any, is provided for your representative(s):

  (i) by your organisation or group? (please give details)

  (ii) by the NHS organisation(s) you are working with? (please give details)

  (iii) by other local/regional/national organisations (e.g. Community Service Volunteers (CSV), Cancerlink, etc.)?

continued opposite

7 What emotional support, if any, is provided for your representative(s):

  (i) by your organisation or group? (please give details)

  (ii) by the NHS organisation(s) you are working with? (please give details)

  (iii) by other local/regional/national organisations (e.g. CSV, Cancerlink, etc.)?

8 What other support, if any, is provided for your representative(s):

  (i) by your organisation or group? (please give details)

  (ii) by the NHS organisation(s) you are working with? (please give details)

  (iii) by other local/regional/national organisations (e.g. CSV, Cancerlink, etc.)?

9 What, if any, have been the specific benefits to your group or organisation of being involved?

10 In which of the following methods for involving users have representatives from your organisation or group been asked to take part? (please tick all that apply)

☐ Focus groups   ☐ Citizen juries   ☐ Postal questionnaires

☐ Face-to-face questionnaires   ☐ Telephone questionnaires   ☐ Public meetings

☐ Complaints procedure   ☐ Health panel   ☐ Representatives on committees

☐ Interviews   ☐ Others (please list)

11 Of the above methods, which have you found to be most effective for involving your representative(s) and why?

continued overleaf

12 When users from your organisation or group take part in NHS user involvement activities, whose views do you expect them to represent? (please tick those which apply)

☐ Their own views

☐ The views of people in similar circumstances

☐ The views of the wider public

☐ The views of your group or organisation

13 With which aspect(s) of NHS cancer services has your group or organisation been involved? (please tick all that apply)

☐ Individual patient care	☐ Service planning	☐ Service review
☐ Resource allocation	☐ Standard setting	☐ Recruitment/ staffing issues
☐ Research	☐ Education/training	☐ Patient needs assessment
☐ Planning future services	☐ Monitoring	☐ Evaluating existing services
☐ Audit	☐ Fundraising	☐ Patient information literature
☐ Others (please list)		

14 What activities have specifically involved representatives from your organisation in *developing* NHS cancer services? (please give up to three examples)

(i)

(ii)

(iii)

continued opposite

15 What activities have specifically involved representatives from your organisation in *evaluating* NHS cancer services? (please give up to three examples)

(i)

(ii)

(iii)

16 What feedback, if any, has your organisation received from the user involvement activities with which it has participated?

17 How helpful/timely has this feedback been?

Section 3: The importance of user involvement in NHS cancer services

The following set of statements asks you to consider, *from the perspective of your organisation or group,* the importance of user involvement in NHS services. Please tick the one term that best describes the importance of user involvement for your organisation.

1 Users' views can be incorporated into organisation plans, but *overall decision-making responsibility rests with managers.*

☐ Agree strongly ☐ Agree ☐ Disagree ☐ Disagree strongly

2 Users' views can be incorporated into organisational plans, but *overall decision-making responsibility rests with clinicians.*

☐ Agree strongly ☐ Agree ☐ Disagree ☐ Disagree strongly

3 Users' views can best be incorporated through *shared decision making with managers.*

☐ Agree strongly ☐ Agree ☐ Disagree ☐ Disagree strongly

4 Users' views can best be incorporated through *shared decision making with clinicians.*

☐ Agree strongly ☐ Agree ☐ Disagree ☐ Disagree strongly

5 Users' views can best be incorporated through *shared decision making with managers and clinicians.*

☐ Agree strongly ☐ Agree ☐ Disagree ☐ Disagree strongly

6 Users should have overall responsibility for decision making *supported by managers.*

☐ Agree strongly ☐ Agree ☐ Disagree ☐ Disagree strongly

7 Users should have overall responsibility for decision making *supported by clinicians.*

☐ Agree strongly ☐ Agree ☐ Disagree ☐ Disagree strongly

8 Users should have overall responsibility for decision making *supported by clinicians and managers.*

☐ Agree strongly ☐ Agree ☐ Disagree ☐ Disagree strongly

9 Users can *contribute to 'service development' by providing their views and feedback.*

☐ Agree strongly ☐ Agree ☐ Disagree ☐ Disagree strongly

10 Users can *contribute to 'service evaluation' by providing their views and feedback.*

☐ Agree strongly ☐ Agree ☐ Disagree ☐ Disagree strongly

Section 4: Further comments about user involvement in your own organisation or group

Are there any other comments about user involvement that you would like to add? (including any ways in which users are involved in your own organisation or group)

Please provide the details of anyone else in your organisation to whom it would be appropriate to send this questionnaire, if anyone.

Name:
Role/job title:
Contact telephone no.:

Name:
Role/job title:
Contact telephone no.:

Name:
Role/job title:
Contact telephone no.:

Thank you for your time and expertise. Please could you return this form in the envelope provided.

If you have any questions about the research or would like to make further comments, please contact:

Michail Sanidas
ASWCS
Kings Square House
Kings Square
Bristol
BS2 8EE

Direct line: 0117 900 2317
Fax no: 0117 900 2388
Email: michail.sanidas@userm.avonhealth.swest.nhs.uk

B: Nominal group technique scoring sheets

Nominal group technique: facilitator's score sheet (rounds 1 and 2)

This score sheet can be used to aggregate the participants' votes during round 1 or round 2 of the Delphi technique.

In the second column, the facilitator inserts the preferences of the participants, while the final ranking (fourth column) is based on the total score (third column).

Below is an example of a first-round Delphi in which four participants have to choose their top 10 statements from a total of 12 statements.

Statement	Individual scores				Total score	Ranking
1	7	5	6		18	7
2	4	8	9	6	27	2
3	9	10	1	9	29	1
4	5	6	10	5	26	3
5	10		3	10	23	5
6	1	4	8	4	17	8
7	8				8	10
8	2	1	4	8	15	9
9	6	9	7	3	25	4
10		7	5	7	19	6
11	3	3		2	7	
12		2	2	1	5	

Nominal group technique: participant's score sheet (round 1)

Two different types of scoring aids can be used during this stage.

In the first method, participants can be given 10 cards. On each card they are asked to write the statement number in the middle of the card, and the score (out of 10) for that statement in the top right-hand corner as follows:

	Score (out of 10)
Statement number	

Alternatively, a scoring sheet can be used, on which participants have to indicate their top 10 preferences. A scoring card could look like this once it has been filled in:

Statement number	Your score
5	10
13	9
7	8
8	7
6	6
22	5
11	4
19	3
10	2
2	1

Nominal group technique: participant score sheet (round 2)

During the second stage of the Delphi technique, participants are given a scoring card on which the statements are listed in descending order. Participants are asked to give a score out of 100 for each statement. A scoring sheet could look like this once it has been filled in:

Statement ranking	Statement	Your score (out of 100)
1	The aim of user involvement is to improve cancer services	87
2	Users should be able to be involved in decisions about their care	65
3	To get users involved, there must be a willingness of professionals to accept users' participation	89
4	There should be a good organisational system to support user involvement	99
5	It should be clear to everyone why they are taking part in user involvement	78
6	It is important to give feedback to users who have been consulted	90
7	All users' communication needs should be addressed, including those arising from language, physical and psychological difficulties	60
8	Information about opportunities for user involvement should be provided as part of general information on cancer services	32
9	There should be a variety of methods available that meet users' practical and emotional needs	97
10	It may not always be possible to accommodate users' expectations. There is a need to balance 'wish lists' with reality	27

C: Delphi questionnaire 1

Developing a consensus statement for user involvement in cancer services

Below is a list of statements made by several groups in response to the question 'What are the key issues to consider when involving users in the development of cancer services?'. We now need to select key statements that will help to guide the development of user involvement. Please state how much you agree or disagree with each statement by circling a number on the scale from 5 (agree strongly) through 3 (neither agree nor disagree) to 1 (disagree strongly).

Who are users? Who should be involved in the development of cancer services?

1.1 Patients should be given the opportunity to be involved in the development of cancer services.   5 4 3 2 1

1.2 When involving patients, it is important to involve their carers as well.   5 4 3 2 1

1.3 User involvement requires liaison with voluntary groups and organisations.   5 4 3 2 1

1.4 There should be opportunities for all citizens to be involved in the development of cancer services.   5 4 3 2 1

What are the aims of user involvement?

2.1 The aim of user involvement is to find out about patient satisfaction with existing cancer services.   5 4 3 2 1

2.2 The aim of user involvement is to improve cancer services.   5 4 3 2 1

2.3 The aim of user involvement is to improve clinical care.   5 4 3 2 1

2.4 Users are entitled to be involved in service development, regardless of the benefits to the service.   5 4 3 2 1

What are the benefits of user involvement?

3.1 User involvement should lead to shared understanding between professionals and users.   5 4 3 2 1

3.2 User involvement should increase the opportunities that users have for obtaining support.   5 4 3 2 1

3.3 User involvement should provide evidence for the evaluation of cancer services.   5 4 3 2 1

The scope of user involvement: how far should it go?

4.1 Users should be involved in setting out priorities for cancer services.   5 4 3 2 1

4.2 Users should be able to be involved in decisions about their care.   5 4 3 2 1

4.3 Users should be involved in decisions about all aspects of cancer services.   5 4 3 2 1

4.4 It may not always be possible to accommodate users' expectations. There is a need to balance 'wish lists' with reality.   5 4 3 2 1

4.5 Users may not have the 'big picture'. User involvement should target areas where they have relevant knowledge and experience.   5 4 3 2 1

4.6 The impact of user involvement on staff satisfaction needs to be considered.   5 4 3 2 1

What resources are needed for user involvement?

5.1 There should be a good organisational system to support user involvement.   5 4 3 2 1

5.2 Users' practical needs, such as transport and access to venues, should be met.   5 4 3 2 1

5.3 Users should be reimbursed for their time when involved in service development.   5 4 3 2 1

5.4 Users should be reimbursed for their costs when involved in service development.   5 4 3 2 1

5.5 Resources for user involvement should be made available to user groups.   5 4 3 2 1

5.6 There should be easily identifiable personnel to offer support to involved users.   5 4 3 2 1

How can we develop a culture of user involvement?

6.1 User involvement should be part of the mainstream culture of health and social services.   5 4 3 2 1

6.2 It is important to build trust and break down barriers between professionals and users, including those of status, culture and communication.   5 4 3 2 1

6.3 All those taking part in user involvement need to be non-judgemental, supportive and able to value people's experience.   5 4 3 2 1

6.4 User involvement should be sustainable and not just a 'one-off' exercise.   5 4 3 2 1

6.5 User participation needs to be real and on equal terms, not just lip service.   5 4 3 2 1

6.6 Users should be able to give feedback on the service 5 4 3 2 1
they have received at any point. It should be a
standard expectation of all those involved.
6.7 For user involvement to work, there has to be 5 4 3 2 1
willingness on the part of users to be involved.
6.8 To get users involved, there must be a willingness 5 4 3 2 1
of professionals to accept users' participation.

Information and communication: what are the key issues?

7.1 Information should be clear and accessible, and 5 4 3 2 1
jargon should be avoided.
7.2 All users' communication needs should be 5 4 3 2 1
addressed, including those arising from language,
physical and psychological difficulties.
7.3 It is important to remove status barriers that may 5 4 3 2 1
affect communication between professionals and
service users.
7.4 It should be clear to everyone why they are taking 5 4 3 2 1
part in user involvement.
7.5 It is important not to raise expectations that cannot 5 4 3 2 1
be met. Users need clear information about the
boundaries of user involvement.
7.6 Information about opportunities for user involvement 5 4 3 2 1
should be provided as part of general information on
cancer services.
7.7 In order to be involved, users need to be well 5 4 3 2 1
informed about how cancer services work.
7.8 In order for user involvement to be effective, health 5 4 3 2 1
professionals need to be well informed about how
users may feel.
7.9 Information about user involvement should be 5 4 3 2 1
available at every stage of cancer care.
7.10 Information about user involvement should take 5 4 3 2 1
into account the user's emotional state and how
much information they can cope with.

Including diverse groups: what are the main issues?

8.1 User involvement should include everyone. 5 4 3 2 1
Social class, sex, ethnicity, education and
geographical location should not be barriers
to participation.
8.2 There should be representation of all groups in 5 4 3 2 1
user involvement. This means that there should be
a cross-section of people of different backgrounds,
including social class, sex, ethnicity, education and
geographical location.

8.3 There is a need to make sure that patients with different   5 4 3 2 1
types of cancer are included in user involvement.
8.4 There should be a selection process for users who   5 4 3 2 1
are seeking to be involved in service development.
8.5 There is a need to make sure that involved users   5 4 3 2 1
really do want to be involved.
8.6 There is a need to make sure that the views expressed   5 4 3 2 1
by involved users are representative of the wider group.
8.7 Involved users should be seen as contributing their   5 4 3 2 1
own experiences, not as speaking for their group.
8.8 Users should choose who they want to represent them. 5 4 3 2 1

Methods: how should users be involved?

9.1 Appropriate methods of user involvement are   5 4 3 2 1
needed in order to obtain relevant information
from users.
9.2 There should be a variety of methods available   5 4 3 2 1
that meet users' practical and emotional needs.
9.3 Group-based discussions are a useful way of   5 4 3 2 1
involving users.
9.4 Questionnaires are a useful method of obtaining   5 4 3 2 1
feedback from users.
9.5 There should be an opportunity for one-to-one   5 4 3 2 1
interviews as a method of user involvement.
9.6 Feedback forms should be used more widely and   5 4 3 2 1
effectively to obtain information from users.
9.7 There is a need to ensure confidentiality for users.   5 4 3 2 1
9.8 People who facilitate user involvement should be   5 4 3 2 1
independent and not involved in the care of users.
9.9 There should be an opportunity for users to opt   5 4 3 2 1
out of the process at any stage.

Training for user involvement: what are the key issues?

10.1 Training should be available to users to ensure the   5 4 3 2 1
effectiveness of their involvement.
10.2 Training should be available to staff to enable them   5 4 3 2 1
to be effective in involving users.
10.3 Everyone working with users should have   5 4 3 2 1
up-to-date knowledge about the cancer services
provided by the health authority.
10.4 Everyone involved should be helped to understand   5 4 3 2 1
the emotional issues that affect users.
10.5 GPs need to be kept up to date with user   5 4 3 2 1
involvement in cancer care.

How should users' experiences and needs be recognised?

11.1	There should be emotional support for users when they are participating in user involvement.	5 4 3 2 1
11.2	It is important to recognise the isolation that patients and carers can feel, and to provide appropriate support.	5 4 3 2 1
11.3	It is important to take into account where users are in their 'cancer journey'.	5 4 3 2 1
11.4	It is important to recognise when particular low points occur for patients, and to take this into account in user involvement.	5 4 3 2 1

Feedback and implementation: how can we maximise the impact of user involvement?

12.1	It is important to give feedback to users who have been consulted.	5 4 3 2 1
12.2	There is a need to give feedback to users to establish the effectiveness of their involvement.	5 4 3 2 1
12.3	Users should not be involved unless it is possible to change practice/policy as a result of their input.	5 4 3 2 1
12.4	It is important to give clear information to users about how decisions are made.	5 4 3 2 1
12.5	It is important to put into action the results of users' input.	5 4 3 2 1

Please write any further comments in this box.

[ ]

Please return your completed questionnaire by 4 June 2001 in the FREEPOST envelope provided to:

ASWCS
FREEPOST (SWB1590)
Bristol BS2 8ZZ

Thank you for taking time to complete the questionnaire. Please tick below to indicate whether you are willing to take part in a follow-up questionnaire.

Yes ☐   No ☐

D: Delphi questionnaire 2

Developing a consensus statement for user involvement in cancer services

You recently completed a questionnaire that aimed to identify key priorities for the development of user involvement in cancer services. Many people took part, including service users, voluntary sector representatives, doctors, managers and nurses. A summary of the results is available on request from Michail Sanidas at the address given at the end of this questionnaire.

Below is a table that lists the most popular statements. Everyone was given an opportunity to agree or disagree with each statement. Some statements were supported by everyone. Others have been included because they obtained broad support, although a very small number of individuals may have disagreed with them.

These statements are shown with a number that indicates how highly each of them was ranked by everyone (first, second, third, etc.). We now need to find out whether this ranking reflects individuals' priorities. This will help us to finalise the consensus statement. We would like you to complete the questionnaire, this time indicating your own ranking of the importance of each statement. Your ranking might be the same as the overall ranking, or it might be different.

Part One: ranking statements within themes

Please use the right-hand column to indicate your ranking.

Who are users? Who should be involved in the development of cancer services?

	Overall ranking	Your ranking
Patients should be given the opportunity to be involved in the development of cancer services.	1	
When involving patients, it is important to involve their carers as well.	2	
User involvement requires liaison with voluntary groups and organisations.	3	

What are the aims and benefits of user involvement?

	Overall ranking	Your ranking
The aim of user involvement is to improve cancer services.	1	
The aim of user involvement is to find out about patient satisfaction with existing cancer services.	2	
The aim of user involvement is to improve clinical care.	3	

The scope of user involvement: how far should it go?

	Overall ranking	Your ranking
Users should be able to be involved in decisions about their own care.	1	
It may not always be possible to accommodate users' expectations. There is a need to balance 'wish lists' with reality.	2	
Users may not have the 'big picture'. User involvement should target areas where they have relevant knowledge and experience.	3	

How can we develop a culture of user involvement?

	Overall ranking	Your ranking
To get users involved, there must be a willingness of professionals to accept users' participation.	1	
It is important to build trust and break down barriers between professionals and users, including those of status, culture and communication.	2	
User participation needs to be real and on equal terms, not just lip service.	3	

What resources are needed for user involvement?

	Overall ranking	Your ranking
There should be a good organisational system to support user involvement.	1	
There should be easily identifiable personnel to offer support to involved users.	2	
Users' practical needs, such as transport and access to venues, should be met.	3	

How can we improve information and communication?

	Overall ranking	Your ranking
Information should be clear and accessible, and jargon should be avoided.	1	
All users' communication needs should be addressed, including those arising from language, physical and psychological difficulties.	2	
It is important to remove status barriers that may affect communication between professionals and service users.	3	

Information and communication: more key issues

	Overall ranking	Your ranking
It should be clear to everyone why they are taking part in user involvement.	1	
It is important not to raise expectations that cannot be met. Users need clear information about the boundaries of user involvement.	2	
Information about opportunities for user involvement should be provided as part of general information on cancer services.	3	

Including diverse groups: what are the main issues?

	Overall ranking	Your ranking
User involvement should include everyone. Social class, sex, ethnicity, education, geographical location, cancer type and illness stage should not be barriers to participation.	1	
There is a need to make sure that patients with different types of cancer are included in user involvement.	2	
There should be equal representation of all groups in user involvement. This means that there should be a cross-section of people of different backgrounds, including social class, sex, ethnicity, education and geographical location.	3	

Methods: how should users be involved?

	Overall ranking	Your ranking
There should be a variety of methods available that meet users' practical and emotional needs.	1	
There is a need to ensure confidentiality for users.	2	
Appropriate methods of user involvement are needed in order to obtain relevant information from users.	3	

Training for user involvement: what are the key issues?

	Overall ranking	Your ranking
Everyone involved should be helped to understand the emotional issues that affect users.	1	
GPs need to be kept up to date with user involvement.	2	
Training should be available to staff to enable them to be effective in involving users.	3	

How should users' experiences and needs be recognised?

	Overall ranking	Your ranking
It is important to recognise when particular low points occur for patients and to take this into account in user involvement.	1	
It is important to recognise where people are in their 'cancer journey'.	2	
It is important to recognise the isolation that patients and carers can feel, and to provide appropriate support.	3	

Feedback and implementation: how can we maximise the impact of user involvement?

	Overall ranking	Your ranking
It is important to give feedback to users who have been consulted.	1	
There is a need to give feedback to users to establish the effectiveness of their involvement.	2	
It is important to put into action the results of users' input.	3	

Part Two: ranking the consensus statements

Below is a list of nine statements. These are the statements that received universal support. No one disagreed with these statements at all, and they will all be included in the final consensus statement. However, we wish to find out which statements represent the most important priorities.

From the statements below, please choose the five that are most important to you and rank them from 1 to 5 (where 1 = the most important statement).

Statement	Rank
The aim of user involvement is to improve cancer services.	
Users should be able to be involved in decisions about their care.	
It should be clear to everyone why they are taking part in user involvement.	
To get users involved, there must be a willingness of professionals to accept users' participation.	
It is important to give feedback to users who have been consulted.	
All users' communication needs should be addressed, including those arising from language, physical and psychological difficulties.	
There should be a good organisational system to support user involvement.	
Information about opportunities for user involvement should be provided as part of general information on cancer services.	
There should be a variety of methods available that meet users' practical and emotional needs.	

Please write any further comments in this box.

Please return your completed questionnaire by 23 July 2001 in the FREEPOST envelope provided to:

ASWCS
FREEPOST (SWB1590)
Bristol BS2 8ZZ

Thank you for taking time to complete the questionnaire. Please tick below to indicate whether you would like to receive a copy of the final consensus statement.

Yes ☐   No ☐

E: A consensus statement for user involvement in cancer services

- The aim of user involvement is to improve cancer services.
- Users should be able to be involved in decisions about their care.
- To get users involved, there must be a willingness of professionals to accept users' participation.
- There should be a good organisational system to support user involvement.
- It should be clear to everyone why they are taking part in user involvement.
- It is important to give feedback to users who have been consulted.
- All users' communication needs should be addressed, including those arising from language, physical and psychological difficulties.
- Information about opportunities for user involvement should be provided as part of general information on cancer services.
- There should be a variety of methods available that meet users' practical and emotional needs.

F: A consensus statement: long version

Developing and evaluating best practice for user involvement in cancer services

1 Aims and scope of user involvement

1.1 **The aim of user involvement is to improve cancer services.**

1.2 **Users should be able to be involved in decisions about their own care.**

1.3 The aim of user involvement is to find out about patient satisfaction with existing cancer services.

1.4 It may not always be possible to accommodate users' expectations. There is a need to balance 'wish lists' with reality.

2 Who should be involved in the development of cancer services?

2.1 Patients should be given the opportunity to be involved in the development of cancer services.

2.2 When involving patients, it is important to involve their carers as well.

2.3 User involvement should include everyone. Social class, sex, ethnicity, education, geographical location, cancer type and illness stage should not be barriers to participation.

2.4 There is a need to make sure that patients with different types of cancer are included in user involvement.

3 Developing a culture of user involvement

3.1 **To get users involved, there must be a willingness of professionals to accept users' participation.**

3.2 It is important to build trust and break down barriers between professionals and users, including those of status, culture and communication.

3.3 It is important to recognise when particular low points occur for patients and to take this into account in user involvement.

3.4 It is important to recognise where people are in their 'cancer journey'.

3.5 *User participation needs to be real and on equal terms, not just lip service.*

4 Resources, strategies and methods of user involvement

4.1 **There should be a good organisational system to support user involvement.**

4.2   **There should be a variety of methods available that meet users'
practical and emotional needs.**

4.3   There should be easily identifiable personnel to offer support to
involved users.

4.4   There is a need to ensure confidentiality for users.

4.5   Everyone involved should be helped to understand the
emotional issues that affect users.

4.6   Training should be available to staff to enable them to be
effective in involving users.

4.7   *Appropriate methods of user involvement are needed in order to obtain
relevant information from users.*

5 Information, communication and feedback

5.1   **It should be clear to everyone why they are taking part in user
involvement.**

5.2   **It is important to give feedback to users who have been
consulted.**

5.3   **All users' communication needs should be addressed, including
those arising from language, physical and psychological
difficulties.**

5.4   **Information about opportunities for user involvement should be
provided as part of general information on cancer services.**

5.5   Information should be clear and accessible, and jargon should be
avoided.

5.6   It is important not to raise expectations that cannot be met. Users
need clear information about the boundaries of user
involvement.

5.7   There is a need for feedback to users to establish the effectiveness
of their involvement.

5.8   *It is important to remove status barriers that may affect communication
between professionals and service users.*

Bold = universal support was given to these statements.
Italic = ranked third by sample, but strongly supported by one group.
All other statements were ranked first or second by sample.

G: Criteria for evaluating user involvement

A Aims and scope of user involvement

1 The aims of any user involvement initiative are clearly identified at the outset.
2 There are opportunities for users to be involved in service evaluation.
3 There are opportunities for users to be involved in service development.
4 There is a clear definition of 'the user' in relation to any particular initiative.

B Systematic approach to user involvement

5 User involvement activities are undertaken in a regular way as part of a cycle of work.
6 User involvement methods are clearly justified on the basis of the aims of the exercise.
7 User involvement methods take into account users' needs and preferences.
8 User involvement methods are accepted as valid approaches to data collection.
9 Data generated from user involvement processes are managed in an appropriate fashion.

C Resources for user involvement

10 Appropriate resources, including staff time, are made available in order to ensure the success of user involvement initiatives.
11 Appropriate reimbursement is made for involved users' costs (e.g. travel, childcare, time, etc.).

D Information and communication

12 Information about opportunities for user involvement is made available to all service users as part of general information about cancer services.
13 Informed consent for participation is sought from involved users prior to their participation.
14 Communication needs that users may have, including language and literacy needs as well as physical needs, are identified and addressed.
15 Appropriate information about issues on which users are consulted is made available in appropriate formats to all participants.

E Training and support

16 There is evidence of user involvement training for users.
17 There is evidence of user involvement training for staff.
18 There are identified support mechanisms for involved service users.
19 There is support for staff who are undertaking or affected by user involvement initiatives.

F Representation and inclusion

20 There is evidence of a structured approach to recruitment, with attention being paid to groups that are seen as hard to reach.
21 Demographic factors (e.g. socioeconomic background, age, gender, ethnicity, etc.) are taken into account with regard to user recruitment and interpretation of user involvement data.
22 Disease-specific characteristics (including stage and type of treatment) are taken into account with regard to user recruitment and interpretation of user involvement data.
23 User involvement activities include consultation and participation with appropriate voluntary organisations.
24 There is agreement, input and involvement from different categories of staff, including clinicians, nurses, allied health professionals and receptionists/secretaries.

G Power and control

25 There is evidence that user involvement is about user decision making rather than simply 'consumer' preference.
26 There are clear mechanisms to ensure that all staff are 'on board' in terms of responding and being willing to participate in user involvement activities.
27 If users are to be excluded from service evaluation, there is a clear rationale for this.
28 If users are to be excluded from service development, there is a clear rationale for this.

H Evidence of change

29 There is regular review of the impact of user involvement on changes in service delivery.
30 There are clear mechanisms for documenting change in service delivery in response to user involvement activities.

I Feedback and follow-up

31 Appropriate feedback is given to involved users about specific responses to those activities in which they have participated.

32 There is appropriate evaluation of the changes made in response to user involvement in the light of information about the outcomes sought by users.

33 There is appropriate evaluation of all those who participated in user involvement activities. This should address users' satisfaction with both the process and the outcomes.

H: A user involvement questionnaire

Below is the text that introduces the questionnaire.

User involvement in cancer services

This questionnaire asks you to tell us about your experience of NHS cancer services and any part you have played in helping to evaluate or develop those services. These activities, often termed *user involvement*, may consist of asking patients and carers for their views on the service, or asking them to help make decisions about new developments. Your feedback will help us to advise on how to ensure that together, doctors, health professionals and users of cancer services are all involved in developing the best possible cancer services.

Your experience is unique, and you are an expert on your own cancer care. This means that your views are essential if we are to understand how to make cancer services better. The answers you give us will be kept completely confidential, and you will not be identified to anyone who is providing clinical care or support.

Section 1: Your details

Please give us some basic background information about yourself.

1 In what year were you born?   19___

2 What is your ethnic origin? (*please tick or write the answer*)

☐ White ☐ Black African ☐ Chinese ☐ Black Caribbean
☐ Pakistani ☐ Bangladeshi ☐ Indian ☐ Other ....

3 Where do you live? (*please tick or write the answer*)

☐ City ☐ Town ☐ Village ☐ Rural area ☐ Other ....

4 Tell us about your current or last job. (*please tick or write the answer*)

☐ Student ☐ Full-time work ☐ Part-time work ☐ Unemployed
☐ Retired

Job title: ....

5 Who do you live with? (tick all that apply)

☐ Alone ☐ Husband ☐ Wife ☐ Partner ☐ Parents
☐ Daughter ☐ Son ☐ Other person

6 What job does your husband/wife/partner do? (*if applicable*)

Job title: ☐ Full-time ☐ Part-time

7 Describe yourself (*please tick*)

☐ Someone who had cancer ☐ Someone who has cancer

8 With what type of cancer were you diagnosed?

9 When was it originally diagnosed? (month/year)

10 Which hospital(s) provide(d) treatment? (*if applicable*)

11 Which NHS treatments have you had? (*tick all that apply*)

☐ Surgery ☐ Chemotherapy ☐ Radiotherapy
☐ Palliative treatment ☐ Hospice care ☐ Drugs/medication
☐ Psychological/counselling ☐ Other

continued opposite

12 What was your most recent cancer treatment?

When was this? (month/year)

13 Which complementary therapies have you had? (*tick all that apply*)

☐ Aromatherapy   ☐ Reflexology   ☐ Massage
☐ Shiatsu   ☐ Acupuncture   ☐ Relaxation/visualisation
☐ Reiki healing   ☐ Spiritual healing   ☐ Homeopathy
☐ None   ☐ Other

Section 2: User involvement in cancer services

The next set of questions asks you about your experience of helping to improve cancer services.

2.1 Did you join a support group for any of the following reasons? (*please tick all that apply*)

☐ Did not join a   ☐ To meet other people   ☐ To pressurise for better
support group   with cancer   cancer services
☐ Because I was   ☐ For personal   ☐ To help support
asked to   support   others
☐ To give something   ☐ To obtain   ☐ To get better care for
back   information   my cancer
☐ None   ☐ Other ....

2.2 Have you been involved in any other community organisations? (*please tick all that apply*)

☐ Sports club   ☐ Local politics   ☐ Church/religious
group   ☐ Volunteering   ☐ Continuing education
☐ School   ☐ None   ☐ Other ....

2.3 Have you participated in any of the following methods of improving cancer services? (*please tick all that apply*)

☐ None (if none, please go directly to Section 3)
☐ Focus groups   ☐ Citizen juries   ☐ Questionnaires   ☐ Public meetings
☐ Health panel   ☐ Complaints   ☐ National cancer   ☐ Representative
☐ Drug trial/   procedure   patients survey   on committee
research   ☐ Fundraising   ☐ User involvement group
☐ Other ....

continued overleaf

2.4 Please tell us more about the items you ticked in the previous question (2.3). What was your experience of being involved in evaluating and/or developing cancer services? (please give details)

Which was your most recent experience?

The following questions ask you *only about your most recent* experience of user involvement in cancer services.

2.5 When were you most recently involved in the evaluation and improvement of cancer services? (*please tick only one*)

☐ As soon as diagnosed   ☐ Within 1 year of diagnosis
☐ 1–2 years after diagnosis   ☐ 2–3 years after diagnosis
☐ 3–4 years after diagnosis   ☐ 4–5 years after diagnosis
☐ More than 5 years after diagnosis   ☐ Other ....

2.6 With hindsight, in your opinion when would have been the best time for you to be involved in the evaluation and improvement of cancer services? (*please tick only one*)

☐ As soon as diagnosed   ☐ Within 1 year of diagnosis
☐ 1–2 years after diagnosis   ☐ 2–3 years after diagnosis
☐ 3–4 years after diagnosis   ☐ 4–5 years after diagnosis
☐ More than 5 years after diagnosis   ☐ At all times
☐ Other ....

2.7 Why did you get involved? (*please tick all that apply*)

☐ To improve local cancer services   ☐ Because I was asked to
☐ To get better care for my cancer   ☐ To pressurise for change
☐ To give something back services   ☐ To have a say in local cancer
☐ Other ....

2.8 Thinking about your most recent involvement, how did you receive information about becoming involved? (*please tick all that apply*)

☐ Leaflets   ☐ Local television   ☐ Discussion with health
☐ Poster   ☐ Complaint form   professional
☐ Local paper   ☐ Local radio   ☐ Discussion with other user(s)
☐ Feedback/suggestion form   ☐ Other ....

continued opposite

2.9 Thinking about your most recent involvement, with which aspect(s) of NHS cancer services were you involved? (*please tick all that apply*)

☐ My own care
☐ Research
☐ Sharing out resources for cancer services
☐ Patient information leaflets
☐ Don't know

☐ Planning cancer services
☐ Setting standards
☐ Helping with education/training
☐ Fundraising
☐ Reviewing current cancer services

☐ Recruiting staff
☐ Evaluating existing services
☐ Helping to provide care (e.g. volunteering)
☐ Other

2.10 In your most recent involvement, were you offered any of the following forms of support? (*please tick all that apply*)

☐ Pay for travel expenses
☐ Pay for time
☐ None

☐ Provide with transport
☐ Training
☐ Other(s)

☐ Provide with or pay for childcare
☐ Emotional support

2.11 What happened as a result of your most recent involvement? (*please give details*)

2.12 What other forms of support would have helped you to be involved? (*please tick all that apply*)

☐ Pay for travel expenses
☐ Pay for time
☐ I was happy with what I received

☐ Provide with transport
☐ Training
☐ Other(s)

☐ Provide with or pay for childcare
☐ Emotional support

continued overleaf

Below are a series of statements. You should answer each statement by itself. This is not a test of what you know. There are no right or wrong answers. We are only interested in your opinions or impression. Please circle only one number for each statement.

Thinking about my most recent involvement:	Strongly agree	Agree	Neither agree nor disagree	Disagree	Strongly disagree
2.13 It is likely to improve cancer services.	1	2	3	4	5
2.14 It was easy for me to be involved.	1	2	3	4	5
2.15 I was given appropriate feedback on the results of my involvement.	1	2	3	4	5
2.16 I found my experience personally rewarding.	1	2	3	4	5
2.17 I felt that my involvement was welcomed.	1	2	3	4	5
2.18 The information about my most recent involvement was easy to understand.	1	2	3	4	5

2.19 What was the *most* rewarding aspect of your most recent involvement?

2.20 What was the *least* rewarding aspect of your most recent involvement?

continued opposite

Section 3: No involvement in evaluating and developing cancer services

This set of questions is for those people who *were not* involved in the evaluation and development of cancer services.

3.1 Some people have suggested the following reasons *for not being involved in the evaluation and improvement of cancer services*. Did any of these apply to you? (*please tick all that apply*)

☐ Was not asked   ☐ Did not have time   ☐ Physically unable
☐ Too distressing   ☐ Too far to travel   ☐ Not my responsibility
☐ Have dependents   ☐ Do not have the   ☐ Emotionally unable
☐ Might negatively   energy   ☐ It would make no
   affect my treatment ☐ I was/am involved   difference
☐ Not interested   ☐ Not given any   ☐ Other(s) ....
☐ Lack of confidence   information about
                          involvement

3.2 Would you like to be involved in the evaluation and improvement of cancer services in the following ways? (*tick all that apply*)

☐ Informal discussions with   ☐ User representative on a local
   NHS staff   NHS committee
☐ Through existing voluntary   ☐ A representative in a user
   organisations   involvement group
☐ Taking part in drug trials/research ☐ Taking part in other research
☐ NHS cancer service open   ☐ Generally interested, but don't
   meetings   know how
☐ Do not wish to be involved

3.3 Would you be willing to be involved in the evaluation and improvement of cancer services in the future using any of the following methods? (*please tick all that apply*)

☐ Focus groups   ☐ Interviews   ☐ Representative on local
☐ Public meetings   ☐ Fundraising   NHS committee
☐ Complaints procedure ☐ Would not want   ☐ National cancer patient
☐ Health panel   to be involved   survey
☐ Citizen juries   ☐ Questionnaires   ☐ Other(s)

3.4 When would be the best time for you to be involved in the evaluation and improvement of cancer services? (*please tick only one*)

☐ As soon as diagnosed   ☐ Within 1 year of diagnosis
☐ 1–2 years after diagnosis   ☐ 2–3 years after diagnosis
☐ 3–4 years after diagnosis   ☐ 4–5 years after diagnosis
☐ More than 5 years after diagnosis ☐ At all times
☐ Other(s) ....

continued overleaf

Please go on to Section 4

Section 4: General satisfaction with cancer services

Below are a series of statements. This is not a test of what you know. There are no right or wrong answers. We are only interested in your opinions or best impression. Please *circle only one number* for each statement.

	Strongly agree	Agree	Neither agree nor disagree	Disagree	Strongly disagree
4.1 I am very satisfied with the cancer care I receive.	1	2	3	4	5
4.2 Doctors are very careful to check everything when examining their patients.	1	2	3	4	5
4.3 I was given enough written information.	1	2	3	4	5
4.4 Doctors always do their best to keep the patient from being anxious.	1	2	3	4	5
4.5 My doctors always treat me with respect.	1	2	3	4	5
4.6 The cancer care I received could have been better.	1	2	3	4	5
4.7 I see the same cancer nurse just about every time I go for cancer care in the hospital.	1	2	3	4	5
4.8 People are usually kept waiting a long time at a clinic to see a cancer doctor (oncologist).	1	2	3	4	5
4.9 Cancer nurses in the hospital hardly ever explain the patient's medical problems to them.	1	2	3	4	5

continued opposite

	Strongly agree	Agree	Neither agree nor disagree	Disagree	Strongly disagree
4.10 District nurses hardly ever explain the patient's medical problems to them.	1	2	3	4	5
4.11 I had an explanation of why X-rays were ordered.	1	2	3	4	5
4.12 Doctors are not thorough enough.	1	2	3	4	5
4.13 It is hard to get an appointment to see a cancer doctor (surgeon) urgently.	1	2	3	4	5
4.14 People are usually kept waiting a long time to get an appointment to see a cancer doctor (oncologist).	1	2	3	4	5
4.15 District nurses are not thorough enough.	1	2	3	4	5
4.16 Macmillan nurses hardly ever explain the patient's medical problems to them.	1	2	3	4	5
4.17 People are usually kept waiting a long time at a clinic to see a cancer doctor (surgeon).	1	2	3	4	5
4.18 My GP is a good source of information.	1	2	3	4	5
4.19 Cancer services are conveniently located.	1	2	3	4	5
4.20 Nurses always do their best to keep the patient from being anxious.	1	2	3	4	5
4.21 The district nurses always treat me with respect.	1	2	3	4	5
4.22 I did not receive good cancer care from my GP.	1	2	3	4	5

continued overleaf

	Strongly agree	Agree	Neither agree nor disagree	Disagree	Strongly disagree
4.23 It is hard to get an appointment to see a cancer doctor (oncologist) urgently.	1	2	3	4	5
4.24 I am worried or concerned about what might happen in the future.	1	2	3	4	5
4.25 I was always told what to expect during treatment.	1	2	3	4	5
4.26 Macmillan nurses are not thorough enough.	1	2	3	4	5
4.27 People are usually kept waiting a long time to get an appointment to see a cancer doctor (surgeon).	1	2	3	4	5
4.28 The cancer clinic was clean.	1	2	3	4	5
4.29 Doctors hardly ever explain the patient's medical problems to them.	1	2	3	4	5
4.30 Cancer nurses in the hospital are not thorough enough.	1	2	3	4	5
4.31 I was told who else I could contact if I needed help when I was at home.	1	2	3	4	5
4.32 I am worried or concerned about the fact I have cancer.	1	2	3	4	5
4.33 The cancer nurses in the hospital always treat me with respect.	1	2	3	4	5
4.34 I am having no difficulty coping with my emotions to do with my cancer.	1	2	3	4	5
4.35 I see the same doctor just about every time I go for cancer care.	1	2	3	4	5
4.36 The cancer clinic was comfortable.	1	2	3	4	5
4.37 A specialist doctor was called when necessary.	1	2	3	4	5
4.38 I can find help if I have a medical question.	1	2	3	4	5

continued opposite

Section 5: Further comments about user involvement

Do you have any other comments about user involvement that you would like to add?

Thank you for your time and expertise. Please could you return this form in the envelope provided. If you have any questions about this research or would like to make further comments, please contact:

Michail Sanidas
ASWCS
Kings Square House
Kings Square
Bristol BS2 8EE

Direct line: 0117 900 2317
Fax no: 0117 900 2388
Email: michail.sanidas@userm.avonhealth.swest.nhs.uk

This research project incorporates a number of different research methods.

Would you be willing to let us contact you again for another part of the research?

Yes ☐   No ☐

If Yes, please give your contact details below:

Name:

Address:

Contact telephone no.:

Index